RHEUMATIC FEVER

Second Edition

Rheumatic Fever
Second Edition

ANGELO TARANTA, MD
Professor of Medicine, New York Medical College
Chief of Medicine, Cabrini Medical Center
New York City, New York, USA

MILTON MARKOWITZ, MD
Professor of Pediatrics
University of Connecticut School of Medicine
Farmington, Connecticut, USA

KLUWER ACADEMIC PUBLISHERS
DORDRECHT / BOSTON / LONDON

Distributors

for the United States and Canada: Kluwer Academic Publishers, PO Box 358, Accord Station, Hingham, MA 02018-0358, USA
for all other countries: Kluwer Academic Publishers Group, Distribution Center, PO Box 322, 3300 AH Dordrecht, The Netherlands

British Library Cataloguing in Publication Data

Taranta, Angelo
    Rheumatic fever. — 2nd ed.
    1. Man. Rheumatic fever
    I. Title   II. Markowitz, Milton
    616.9'91

Library of Congress Cataloging-in-Publication Data

Taranta, Angelo
    Rheumatic fever / Angelo Taranta, Milton Markowitz. — 2nd ed.
        p.   cm.
    Includes bibliographies and index
    ISBN-13: 978-94-010-7060-7   e-ISBN-13: 978-94-009-1261-8
    DOI: 10.1007/978-94-009-1261-8
    1. Rheumatic fever. I. Markowitz, Milton, 1918–   . II. Title.
    [DNLM: 1. Rheumatic Fever.   WC 220 T177r]
    RC182.R4T28 1988
    616.9'91 — dc19
    DNLM/DLC
    for Library of Congress
88-8450 CIP

Copyright

Published in the United Kingdom by Kluwer Academic Publishers, PO Box 55, Lancaster, UK.

Kluwer Academic Publishers BV incorporates the publishing programmes of D. Reidel, Martinus Nijhoff, Dr W. Junk and MTP Press.

Typeset by Lasertext Limited, Stretford, Manchester, England

Contents

Foreword

Today rheumatic fever is still the most common cause of heart disease in children and young adults in developing countries. This disease is typically associated with poverty, in particular with poor housing, overcrowding and inadequate medical care. Rheumatic fever has almost disappeared from economically developed countries; this trend has paralleled improvements in standards of living. However, the recent resurgence of rheumatic fever in middle-class families in the U.S.A. has re-emphasized the importance of this disease in the developed countries as well.

Prevention and control of rheumatic fever and rheumatic heart disease is an important part of the WHO cardiovascular disease program. Based on earlier WHO experience, and on the magnitude of the problem, it was realized that concerted action was needed to combat this significant cause of cardiovascular morbidity and mortality. The present program has been developed on the principle that sound knowledge and reliable technology already exist for implementing community programs for the prevention and control of rheumatic fever and rheumatic heart disease with the intention of extending activities toward nationwide coverage. The first edition of this book was an excellent instrument to assist in the control of this disease. The present volume with dissemination of knowledge to health personnel will contribute to closing the gap between knowledge and implementation and it links with WHO's endeavors in prevention and control of rheumatic fever and rheumatic heart disease.

May I express the wish and hope that this book will be read by all doctors and other health professionals involved in the prevention and control of rheumatic fever and rheumatic heart disease.

SIEGFRIED BOTHIG, M.D.
Chief, Cardiovascular Diseases
World Health Organization

Acknowledgment

The authors wish to thank Jean Anderson, Betty Swanson and Jane Mbeo for their excellent typing of the manuscript, and for their forbearance and good humor. We wish also to thank Michele L. Santangelo and Dr Isha Bhattacharyya for their editorial review of the manuscript.

Preface to the 1981 edition

Why we have written this book

When we were very young, one of us in Europe, the other in North America, rheumatic fever loomed large among the anxieties of lay people and the interests of physicians. At home we heard stories of relatives and friends killed by the disease, of marriages that did not take place because the bride-to-be was found to have had rheumatic fever, and of vocations changed because mitral stenosis interfered with them. Later, after one of us had emigrated to America, we both worked, separately, in specialized chronic hospitals/convalescent homes for children with rheumatic fever, in New York (Irvington House) and in Baltimore (Happy Hills) – hospitals that do not exist any more, not because there is no money to support them, but because there are no patients to fill them. We closed the hospitals and did other things.

Thus, viewed from our front porch, the rheumatic fever story has just about ended; not fully understood, if the truth be told, but controlled nevertheless. From a less narrow perspective, however, we know that the story is altogether different. Most children of the 1980s do not live in Europe or in North America. They live in Asia, in Africa, and in Latin America or, more generally, in what is loosely referred to as the Third World, the developing countries, or the emerging nations. We have traveled many times to these countries and we know that rheumatic fever is still alive and kicking there. Obviously, a gap exists between what could be and what is.

We have written this book to help in closing this gap. We have written it for the medical student and the young physician (young in heart at least!) and for that semi-mythical personage, the health planner; more generally, for the health worker interested in this problem, regardless of the specific previous training. We hope that our readers will be attentive, but also critical. Real progress will be achieved not by repeating, parrot-like, what we have done in the West (we need not build chronic hospitals for rheumatic fever!), but by picking from our experience and knowledge what can be useful elsewhere.

ix

Preface to the 1989 edition

Why a second edition now?

Seven years, as Thomas Mann once wrote, is a goodly span of time, with a mythical ring, lent by the number seven (the seven deadly sins, the seven plagues of Egypt), which neither six nor eight enjoy. That's how long Hans Castorp remained on the Magic Mountain, and that's how long we remained aloof of this little book. But enough new observations have accumulated now to overcome our natural laziness: advances in our knowledge of rheumatic fever, many originating in the developing countries, where so much of the action in rheumatic fever is now; and most recently this historic surprise, the return of rheumatic fever to the U.S.A.

This return, a humbling experience for many of us, has reinforced what we suspected all along: rheumatic fever will not go away for good unless we truly understand and outsmart it. To achieve this aim we must attract new workers to the field, and this second edition has been enlarged with this aim in mind. As a result the book is some 25% larger, but still slim by the usual standards and still made available free of charge, thanks to an educational grant-in-aid from Wyeth-Ayerst International Inc.

It had better remain slim, as we expect it to travel far – to the four corners of the globe, to be exact – or wherever rheumatic fever turns up (or is newly recognized as a problem); and even to our own backyard, where a new generation of physicians is unfamiliar with rheumatic fever, yet has to cope with it now.

The first edition reached, we are told, tens of thousands of readers in 46 countries in its original English-language version, as well as in two Spanish versions. We trust that this second edition will be as lucky, or more. *Bon voyage!*

Chapter 1
DEFINITIONS, HISTORY, AND GEOGRAPHY

Definitions of rheumatic fever and related terms

Rheumatic fever is an acute inflammatory disease which may follow beta-hemolytic, group A streptococcal infections of the throat, but no other infection, and not even streptococcal infections of other sites, such as the skin. Characteristically, it tends to recur. Its name (rheumatic) emphasizes the joints, but it is the heart which makes it important.

Rheumatic fever consists of a number of clinical manifestations, the most common of which is *arthritis*; the most serious, *carditis*; the most curious, *chorea*; the most rare and inconsequential, *subcutaneous nodules* and *erythema marginatum*. They tend to occur together, and may be considered a syndrome ("syndrome = running together"), i.e., they occur in the same patients, at the same time or in close succession, with a much greater frequency than would be expected from chance alone. That's why they are considered part of the same entity*. They may occur singly, however, or in various combinations in any individual patient, though the most common is arthritis and carditis.

"Acute rheumatic fever" is a synonym of rheumatic fever which emphasizes its acute aspects. "Acute articular rheumatism" is another synonym encountered in the European literature. "Inactive rheumatic fever" applies to a patient with a history of rheumatic fever but without evidence of inflammation (it is actually a synonym for "history of rheumatic fever"). "Rheumatic heart disease" denotes the cardiac sequels of rheumatic carditis.

Group A streptococci are one of the causative agents of pharyngitis and *the* causative agent of rheumatic fever. Almost all the group A streptococci are beta-hemolytic; that is, their colonies on blood agar are surrounded by a halo of complete, clear hemolysis, but many beta-hemolytic streptococci are not group A (e.g., groups C and G) and are not important for rheumatic fever. Group A streptococci are sometimes referred to simply as "streptococci" for short, or even, colloquially, as "strep."

---

*By the same token, acute post-streptococcal glomerulonephritis is not considered to be part of the same syndrome: glomerulonephritis, albeit post-streptococcal, does not tend to occur together with rheumatic fever (though occasionally it may).

Brief history of rheumatic fever

Rheumatic fever emerged from the potpourri of "rheumatism" in the seventeenth century, when Guillaume de Baillou in France described it under the name of "acute articular rheumatism" and Thomas Sydenham in England separated it from gout – another acute and recurrent arthritis which, when the attack is over, leaves the joints "as good as new." Neither clinician noted that rheumatic fever affects the heart; and Sydenham, who wrote a masterly description of chorea (therefore called to this day Sydenham's chorea), did not recognize its rheumatic nature. Deformities of the heart valves, first described anatomically by Morgagni in Italy in 1761, were noted to crop up frequently in the autopsies of patients with a history of acute articular rheumatism, but the clinical description of rheumatic heart disease had to await the invention of the stethoscope by Laennec in 1819. By 1886 Cheadle had described the full rheumatic fever syndrome: carditis, polyarthritis, and chorea, as well as subcutaneous nodules and erythema marginatum[1]. Thus, rheumatic fever, as we know it today, resulted from the fitting together of manifestations originally described independently of each other and thought at first to be unrelated (Figure 1.1).

By the beginning of this century Aschoff had described the specific myocardial lesion that bears his name[2] and the connection between a history of a previous sore throat and rheumatic fever was strongly suspected. This perception was reinforced in 1931 by the bacteriologic and epidemiologic studies of Collis in England[3] and of Coburn in the United States[4]. Subsequent immunologic studies more firmly established the relation between group A streptococcal pharyngitis and rheumatic fever. However, the most convincing evidence that streptococcal infections actually cause rheumatic fever

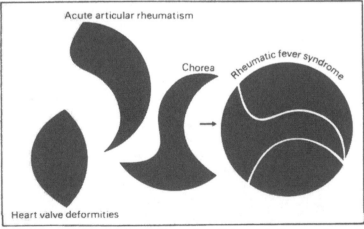

Acute articular rheumatism

Chorea

Rheumatic fever syndrome

Heart valve deformities

Figure 1.1 Historical development of the concept of rheumatic fever syndrome from the fitting together of disease manifestations previously described independently of each other

came from medical intervention. Coburn and Moore in 1939 showed that recurrences of rheumatic fever could be prevented by continual anti-streptococcal medication[5] and a decade later Wannamaker *et al.*[6] demonstrated that adequate treatment of streptococcal pharyngitis with penicillin could prevent first attacks of rheumatic fever. Thus, rheumatic fever emerged as a clinical syndrome with a single etiology, group A beta-hemolytic streptococcal infections of the throat.

After Cheadle's synthetic process took place, analysis followed: a number of entities were recognized that could be confused with rheumatic fever but were differentiated from it on etiologic or clinicopathologic grounds: viral carditis, *Yersinia* arthritis, and mitral valve prolapse, among others (Figure 1.2). As a result, "rheumatic fever" was whittled away but a central core remained which is, we like to think, smaller but more authentic[7].

Another conceptual change is the realization that rheumatic fever itself, the central core, is not homogeneous: one thing is rheumatic fever with carditis and another rheumatic fever without carditis. Attention was called to the latter by the provocative name of post-streptococcal arthritis (instead of rheumatic fever)[8] and by the observation that patients with this disease did well[9], seldom if ever developing rheumatic heart disease on careful follow-up – and even if they had recurrences[9,10]. We prefer to hold on to the traditional term, rheumatic fever, although we emphasize that the specific manifestations in the diagnosis should be identified.

While all these conceptual changes were taking place, the incidence of rheumatic fever was also changing. Although the historical record is sparse, the incidence of rheumatic fever seems to have increased with industrialization and urbanization and then decreased with the subsequent affluence,

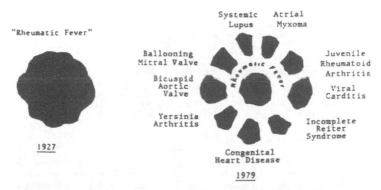

Figure 1.2 The whittling away of rheumatic fever. Many diseases that had not been described or were difficult to diagnose in 1927 (the particular year is arbitrary) were "lumped" together as rheumatic fever (in the presence of fever) or as rheumatic heart disease (in its absence). They are now split off. What remains is a core, smaller but more homogeneous than the original lump

a process completed in the post-industrial West but still developing in the "developing" countries (Figure 1.3).

As will be discussed more fully in the next chapter, availability of penicillin and improvement in the standard of living (especially a decrease of crowding in the home) have been credited for the decrease of rheumatic fever in modern times; yet the most striking decline may have occurred during the 1970s when the standard of living in the U.S. didn't improve and the use of penicillin did not change. One might speculate that rheumatic fever has a "latent period" in its rises and falls in the population at large (just as it does in individual patients after a strep infection) for reasons that are poorly understood.

More recently, unfavorable environmental changes have occurred. As one of us noted 10 years ago, the housing situation in the U.S. has been worsening, with resulting increase in crowding in the home, and this change may have been reflected in the reappearance of rheumatic fever in the mid-1980s[11]. Another "environmental factor", medical care, may also have changed; physicians in the West may have become less compulsive in diagnosing and treating streptococcal infections[12]. This decrease of assiduousness also seems to have had its effect only after a latent period of some years, as if its effect were cumulative as well as additive to the effect of crowding.

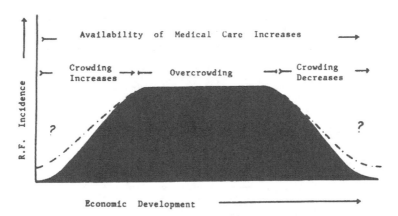

Figure 1.3 Theoretical schema of the evolution of human societies indicates as "development" on the horizontal axis, and the prevalence of rheumatic fever on the vertical axis. In a first state, primitive societies composed of small tribes isolated from each other may be unable to support a multitude of streptococcal types, or to foster their virulence by "passage" through a long chain of hosts; hence no rheumatic fever (perhaps). At the other, or post-industrialized, end of the spectrum, the individuals are isolated again, by large houses and suburbia, and treated. Hence rheumatic fever decreases and perhaps disappears, always ready to bounce back (as it has)

4

Incidence and prevalence

Rheumatic fever occurs in all parts of the world. However, it is difficult to obtain reliable data on the incidence of this disease and the prevalence of its sequel, rheumatic heart disease. There are many published reports, but different diagnostic criteria are often used, the same criteria may be applied differently, the patients studied may not be representative, and the denominator of the population studied is often unknown. Nevertheless, the high proportion of rheumatic heart disease among cardiac patients in developing countries is ample evidence of the impact of rheumatic fever on the health of the people[13].

Incidence

Much of the incidence data that have been published are shown in Table 1.1. Figures as high as 100 per 100,000 population, reported from some of the developing countries, are similar to those from Western countries 75 to 100 years ago[14]. However, even in economically developed countries there are some striking differences in incidence between certain population groups; e.g., Maori, vs. non-Maori in New Zealand and the Samoans vs. Chinese in Hawaii[15,16].

As is apparent from Table 1.1, rheumatic fever is frequently encountered in tropical countries, where it was once believed to be rare (and perhaps it was, when tropical countries were isolated by long and difficult voyages;

Table 1.1 Incidence of acute rheumatic fever in different regions of the world

Locality	Age group (years)	Year	Incidence per 100,000	Reference
Kuwait	5–14	1985	31	17
New Zealand	5–19	1972–83		
Maori			88	15
Non-Maori			9	
Iran	All ages	1972	58–100	13
Cyprus	All ages	1972	27–43	18
Hawaii	4–18	1976–80		16
Chinese			4	
Hawaiian			27	
Samoan			96	
French Polynesia	—	1980–84	72	(unpublished data)
Sri Lanka	5–9	1978	140	13
Baltimore, USA	5–19	1960–64	24	19
		1978–80	0.5	
Denmark	All ages	1962	12	14
Sweden	5–15	1952–56	9	20
		1957–62	2.3	
		1971–80	0.2	

the jets have changed all that)[21]. The recognition of rheumatic fever in these countries in recent times may have come about because there are more and better-trained physicians, and more attention is directed to the health of the local populations than during colonial times. Also, there may be less competition than formerly from such major health problems as smallpox or cholera. However, it is also likely that there has been a real increase in the incidence, for reasons that will be discussed in the next chapter.

The incidence of rheumatic fever in economically developed countries has been changing. It began to decline slowly but steadily beginning after 1900, reaching a level of about 50/100,000 in the mid-1940s. The decline became much more pronounced thereafter, so that by 1980 the annual incidence in several areas of the United States was documented between 0.5 and 2/100,000 population[19,22]. For a time it appeared that in Western countries and Japan, rheumatic fever might soon become a disease of the past. However, the prediction of rheumatic fever's obsolescence turned out to be premature. In 1987, sizeable outbreaks of rheumatic fever in different parts of the United States were reported[23,24]. The patients observed in these outbreaks exhibited the classical manifestations of acute rheumatic fever, and many of them were severely affected. In one outbreak, 19% of the patients were in heart failure and several patients needed valve replacement during the acute attack[23]. Thus, not only is there a resurgence of rheumatic fever, but the disease is as severe as it once was.

Prevalence of rheumatic heart disease

Carditis unaccompanied by other rheumatic manifestations is often asymptomatic, except in its most severe form, and many children with unrecognized rheumatic fever go on to develop progressive valvular heart disease later in life. Thus, as noted earlier, the prevalence of rheumatic heart disease in a population provides a better indicator of the real frequency of rheumatic fever.

Surveys on the prevalence of rheumatic heart disease among schoolchildren have been carried out in a number of countries (Table 1.2). The wide range of figures shown in this table may be due to the methods used in these studies, as well as to genuine differences in the populations surveyed. Nevertheless, in more than half of the countries listed, a high prevalence, from 5 to 20 per 1000 schoolchildren, was found. Even these high figures almost certainly represent an underestimation, since very often rheumatic heart disease is not discovered until adulthood. In countries such as India, Thailand, and Pakistan, rheumatic heart disease makes up between 25 and 40 percent of all cardiac admissions, and there has been no change in these rates of admissions over the past 15 years[25].

6

Table 1.2   Prevalence of RHD among school children in different regions of the world

Locality	Year		Prevalence per 1000	Reference
Africa				
Nigeria	1970		0.3–3	13
Ivory Coast	1985		1.9	26
Soweto, South Africa	1975		6.9	27
Morocco	1973		9.9	17
Egypt	1973		10.0	17
Algeria	1970		15.0	13
Latin America				
Caracas, Venezuela	1976		1.5	28
La Paz, Bolivia	1973		17.0	29
Montevideo, Uruguay	1970		1.0	30
San Juan, Puerto Rico	1980		1.6	31
Brazil	1968–70s		1.0–6.8	13
Asia				
India	1982		9	13
Pakistan	1970s		1.8–11	13
Thailand	1974		1.2–21	13
Taiwan	1971		1.1–1.8	13
Mongolia			3.5	13
China	1979		0.4–2.7	13
Pacific				
Waikald, New Zealand		Maoris	7.6	15
		Non-Maoris	1.0	
French Polynesia	1985		8.0	unpublished data

Community medicine and public health importance

Rheumatic fever is not only of clinical interest but also of public health interest, especially in developing countries. This is so because rheumatic fever is a relatively common disease; it affects preferentially population groups that cannot easily pay for their own medical care, and the disease often has a long-lasting limiting effect on the lifestyle and employability of patients. Even more important, from a public health standpoint, many first attacks and most recurrences of rheumatic fever can be prevented. Prevention can be facilitated by public health or community health efforts; for example, by community health centers, "walk-in" clinics, throat culture services, subsidies for prophylactic medication, diagnostic screening, and school health programs. Such "investments" would diminish the financial burden of repeated hospitalizations and cardiac surgery. In Western countries initiatives for the control of rheumatic fever came from individual physicians and officials of voluntary agencies such as the American Heart Association, who then pressed for government action. The same pattern is

7

emerging in many developing countries but the need for government assistance is more urgent.

References

1. Murphy, G. E. (1943). Evolution of our knowledge of rheumatic fever: historical survey with particular emphasis on rheumatic heart disease. *Bull. Hist. Med.*, **14**, 123
2. Murphy, G. E. (1963). The characteristic rheumatic lesions of striated and of non-striated or smooth muscle cells of the heart. Genesis of the lesions known as Aschoff bodies and those myogenic components known as Aschoff cells or as Anitshckow cells or myocytes. *Medicine*, **42**, 73
3. Collis, W. R. F. (1939). Bacteriology of rheumatic fever. *Lancet*, **2**, 817
4. Coburn, A. F. (1931). *The Factor of Infection in the Rheumatic State*. Baltimore: Williams & Wilkins
5. Coburn, A. F. and Moore, L. V. (1939). The prophylactic use of sulfanilamide in streptococcal respiratory infections with especial reference to rheumatic fever. *J. Clin. Invest.*, **18**, 147
6. Wannamaker, L. W. *et al.* (1951). Prophylaxis of acute rheumatic fever by treatment of the preceding streptococcal infection with various amounts of depot penicillin. *Am. J. Med.*, **10**, 673
7. El-Sadr, W. and Taranta, A. (1979). The spectrum and the specter of rheumatic fever in the 1980s. *Clin. Immunol. Up-Date*, 183
8. Friedberg, C. K. (1959). Rheumatic fever in the adult: criteria and implications. *Circulation*, **19**, 161
9. Roth, I. R., Lingg, C. and Whittemore, A. (1937). Heart disease in children. A. Rheumatic group. I. Certain aspects of the age at onset and of recurrences in 488 cases of juvenile rheumatism ushered in by major clinical manifestations. *Am. Heart J.*, **13**, 36
10. Feinstein, A. R. and Spagnuolo, M. (1960). Mimetic features of rheumatic-fever recurrences. *N. Engl. J. Med.*, **262**, 533
11. Taranta, A. (1979). Rheumatic Fever. In D. J. McCarthy (ed.), *Arthritis and Allied Conditions*. (Philadelphia: Lea and Febiger)
12. Shulman, S. T. (ed.) (1984). *Pharyngitis: management in an era of declining rheumatic fever*. New York: Praeger
13. World Health Organization (1980). Community control of rheumatic heart disease in developing countries: A major public health problem. *WHO Chronicle*, **34**, 336
14. DiSciasco, G. and Taranta, A. (1980). Rheumatic fever in children. *Am. Heart J.*, **99**, 635
15. Talbot, R. G. (1984). Rheumatic fever and rheumatic heart disease in the Hamilton health district, New Zealand: an epidemiologic study. *N.Z. Med. J.*, **97**, 634
16. Chun, L. T. *et al.* (1984). Occurrence and prevention of rheumatic fever among ethnic groups of Hawaii. *Am. J. Dis. Child.*, **138**, 476
17. Rheumatic fever and rheumatic heart disease (1988). Report of a World Health Organization Study Group. *WHO Technical Report Series*. Geneva: World Health Organization (in press)
18. Strasser, T. and Rotta, J. (1973). The control of rheumatic fever and rheumatic heart disease. *WHO Chronicle*, **27**, 49
19. Gordis, L. (1985). The virtual disappearance of rheumatic fever in the United States. *Circulation*, **72**, 1155
20. Schollin, J. and Wesstrom, G. (1985). Acute rheumatic fever in Swedish children. *Acta Paediatr. Scand.*, **74**, 749
21. Markowitz, M. (1981). Observations on the epidemiology and preventability of rheumatic fever in developing countries. *Clin. Ther.*, **4**, 240

22. Land, M.A. and Bisno, A.L. (1983). Acute rheumatic fever: A vanishing disease in suburbia. *J. Am. Med. Assoc.*, **249**, 895
23. Veasey, L. J. *et al.* (1987). Resurgence of acute rheumatic fever in the Intermountain Area of the U.S.A. *N. Engl. J. Med.*, **316**, 421–427
24. Hosier, D. H. *et al.* (1987). Resurgence of acute rheumatic fever. *Am. J. Dis. Child.*, **141**, 730
25. Agarwal, B. L. (1981). Rheumatic heart disease unabated in developing countries. *Lancet*, **2**, 1910
26. Bertrand, E. *et al.* (1979). Etude de la prevalence des cardiopathies, notamment rheumatismales, en milieu scolaire en Côte d'Ivoire. *Bull WHO*, **57**, 471
27. McLaren, M. J. *et al.* (1975). Epidemiology of rheumatic heart disease in black school children of Soweto, Johannesburg. *Br. Med. J.*, **4**, 474
28. Munoz, S. (1986). *Prevention of Rheumatic Fever*. X World Congress of Cardiology. Plenary Session 2. Washington, DC, 14–19 September
29. Ibarnegaray, J. *et al.* (1974). Informe de Bolivia a la V Conferencia Panamericana de Estudio y Prevencion de la Fiebre Reumatica. Buenos Aires, Argentina
30. Portillo, J. M. *et al.* (1974). Data from Uruguay presented at the V Pan-American Rheumatic Fever Conference, Buenos Aires, Argentina
31. Martinez-Pico, A. (1980). Fiebre reumatica aguda en America Latina XI InterAmerican Congress Cardiology Symposium: Rheumatic Fever, San Juan, Puerto Rico, September

Chapter 2
Etiology and epidemiology

The cause of rheumatic fever varies according to the framework in which it is viewed. Within the customary biomedical framework, it is caused by the group A beta-hemolytic streptococci and more specifically by group A beta-hemolytic streptococcal infections of the throat. In a sociomedical framework, rheumatic fever is "caused" by poverty, more specifically by over-crowded housing and inadequate public health. Both frameworks are useful: physicians and other health workers are able to control the disease even in unfavorable environmental conditions; epidemiologists and historians, and even political activists, on the other hand, can understand the variations of rheumatic fever incidence over time and place, and thereby bring it down by improving standards of living and health care.

Streptococcal infections

Group A streptococcal infections of the throat *always* precede the development of rheumatic fever, whether first attacks or recurrences. The most direct evidence which proves that relationship to be causal and not coincidental is provided by prevention. The administration of anti-streptococcal drugs, sulfonamides at first, then oral penicillin, and finally benzathine penicillin by injection, brought about a marked reduction of recurrent attacks; and the treatment of the preceding streptococcal pharyngitis with penicillin (sulfonamides were ineffective in this respect) brought about a marked reduction of first attacks (Table 2.1)[1].

To initiate a rheumatic fever attack, group A streptococci must cause an infection of the pharynx, not just a superficial colonization. Infection can be distinguished from colonization by the appearance of an antibody response to at least one streptococcal antigen; e.g., anti-streptolysin O. The pharyngeal

Table 2.1 Effect of penicillin treatment of acute streptococcal pharyngitis on the incidence of acute rheumatic fever

	No. of patients		
Treatment	Strep. pharyngitis	Rheumatic fever	Attack rate (%)
Penicillin	978	2	0.2
Symptomatic	996	28	2.8

From ref. 1

10

infection need not be symptomatic and may then be detectable only in retrospect by a streptococcal antibody rise.

Growing awareness of the public health importance of rheumatic fever in developing countries stimulated studies of the epidemiology of streptococcal infections in these countries[2-4]. The prevalence of streptococcal carriage in healthy schoolchildren in various countries is shown in Table 2.2. In all of these studies carriage rates were highest in primary schoolchildren. In temperate climates the prevalence is highest during the winter months, while in some tropical countries it is said to be highest during the rainy season.

Table 2.2   Beta-hemolytic streptococcal carriage rates in asymptomatic school children

Country	Years of study	BHS carrier rate (%)
U.S.A.	1961–67	11–28
Philippines	1973–77	25
Japan	1961–67	21
South India	1957–58	42
Indonesia	1977–78	21
Kuwait	1978–79	47

From ref. 7

The incidence of symptomatic streptococcal infections has also been studied (Table 2.3)[5]. The group A streptococcus is the cause of about 20 percent of sore throats in children. The similarity between figures from the United States and two Middle Eastern countries is striking.

Table 2.3   The incidence of group A streptococcal pharyngitis in various countries

Country	No. of patients with pharyngitis	Percentage Group A BHS
Egypt	156	19
Kuwait	465	22
U.S.A.	5500	23

From ref. 7

Surveys have also been done of streptococcal antibodies in asymptomatic schoolchildren. The most extensive survey was carried out by WHO in 1972 on blood samples from seven Asian and African countries. Elevated anti-streptolysin O titers over 200 units in children age 6–10 were found in 18–53 percent (Table 2.4)[6]. These studies indicate that diseases caused by Group A streptococci occur in tropical and subtropical countries and correlate with reports that rheumatic heart disease is prevalent in these countries.

It cannot go unnoticed from the above data that streptococcal infections are much more common than rheumatic fever – that is, the attack rate of rheumatic fever after streptococcal infections is low. Hence the speculations

Table 2.4   Percentage of anti-streptolysin O titers over 200 units in children in various tropical and subtropical countries

Country	Percentage ASO titer over 200 units
Pakistan	18.4
Thailand	17.7
Burma	37.2
Mongolia	52.3
Algeria	36.4
Kenya	40.6
Nigeria	53.3

From ref. 6

about the need for an additional factor or co-factors pertaining to the microorganisms, to the host, or to both. Some streptococcal strains, even though of group A and beta-hemolytic, seem to lack the capacity to elicit rheumatic fever: they are said to be "non-rheumatogenic." Furthermore, in published outbreaks of rheumatic fever in Western countries, including recent ones in the United States, only a limited number of streptococcal serotypes have been implicated (serotypes 3, 5, 18, 19, 24). They are said to be "rheumatogenic."[8]

On the other hand, rheumatogenicity may be due to differences in strains within the same serotype. In analogy with what happens in the laboratory, where we can increase the virulence of a streptococcal strain by "passing" it through a series of mice, increase in virulence may occur also in a closely housed human population which allows rapid passage from throat to throat. In recent times, however, the chain of contagion may be interrupted by treatment with antibiotics, which therefore may alter the nature of the infecting organisms, in addition to just decreasing the number of infections. One such alteration may be the loss of rheumatogenicity.

The evidence tends to favor the concept of rheumatogenicity, but the number, and more importantly, the biologic characteristics of such serotypes, or of different strains of the same serotype, remain to be defined. A better definition of what determines rheumatogenicity may lead to a better understanding of the pathogenesis of rheumatic fever. Furthermore, were it possible to identify rheumatogenic serotypes with certainty, the task of developing an effective streptococcal vaccine would be greatly simplified.

Host factors

All cases of rheumatic fever are preceded by a group A streptococcal pharyngitis but only a small minority of these infections is followed by rheumatic fever. There may be host factors which determine the occurrence of rheumatic fever in a given patient. Some of these factors may pertain to the patient himself, as a number of observations suggest:

(1) Age affects the incidence of rheumatic fever. The peak incidence for both attacks and recurrences is between 5 and 15 years of age (Figure 2.1). However, in developing countries onset between 3 and 5 years of age is not unusual[9]. The age distribution coincides with the high incidence of streptococcal infections in children. Lack of immunity and frequent contact with other children in the home and at school account for the susceptibility of this age group to these infections.

(2) Patients who have already had one attack of the disease tend to have recurrences; i.e., their rheumatic fever attack rate after another streptococcal infection is much higher than in the general population. Also, patients tend to repeat the pattern of their first attack in most subsequent attacks (see Chapter 10).

(3) "Rheumatic fever runs in families," that is, blood relatives of patients with rheumatic fever are more likely to develop it than the general population. This may not mean much since environmental conditions such as poverty and overcrowding also "run in families." Observations in twins are more cogent, showing as they do that monozygotic pairs both develop rheumatic fever seven times more commonly than dizygotic, even though both types of twins share the environment to approximately the same extent (Table 2.5)[10]. Moreover, within the

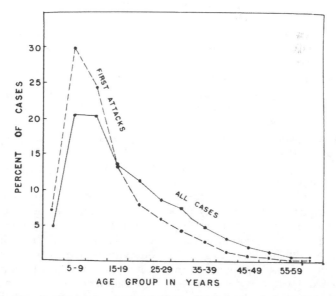

Figure 2.1 The distribution by age group of attacks of rheumatic fever. From Schwentker (1952). In Thomas, L. (ed.) *Rheumatic Fever*. Minneapolis: University of Minnesota Press

Table 2.5   Rheumatic fever in 56 twin pairs

	Concordant pairs	Discordant pairs	Rate (%)
16 monozygotic twin pairs	3	13	18.7
40 dizygotic twin pairs	1	39	2.5

From ref. 10

rheumatic fever syndrome, some individual clinical manifestations of rheumatic fever tend to occur more frequently in the siblings of patients affected by the same manifestation[11]. Therefore there are enough "straws in the wind" to make one think seriously that genetic variation of the host may be an important reason why some patients develop rheumatic fever, and others do not, after what appears to be the same kind of streptococcal infection. Efforts to pin down this postulated "host factor" to a recognizable "marker" have met only with uncertain success in the past. An association of a B-cell alloantigen with susceptibility of rheumatic fever has been reported, but this observation needs additional corroboration[12,13].

Environment

Historically, studies have consistently shown that the incidence of rheumatic fever and the prevalence of rheumatic heart disease are higher among the poor. More recently, however, the return of rheumatic fever in the United States seems to have occurred mostly among the middle class rather than the poor[14].

The relationship between standards of living and the incidence of rheumatic fever is beautifully demonstrated in Figure 2.2, which shows that the decline in rheumatic fever in Western countries began long before the introduction of antimicrobial drugs. This early decline is attributed to improvements in living conditions. More recent examples of this connection can be observed in the decline during the past decade of the prevalence of rheumatic heart disease in the more prosperous Asian countries, such as Japan, Hong Kong and Singapore[15].

A number of observations suggest that, among the manifestations of poverty, crowding is most intimately associated with rheumatic fever. Crowding in the home has a direct relationship with the incidence of rheumatic fever and the prevalence of rheumatic heart disease (Figure 2.3). That this relation is not purely coincidental is suggested by the evidence from the Second World War, when U.S. soldiers, who were well fed and well clothed but lived in overcrowded barracks, developed a high incidence of rheumatic fever. Crowding brings this about because close personal contact facilitates the spread of streptococcal infections, as shown by the relation of the acquisition

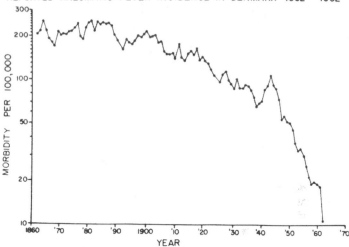

REPORTED RHEUMATIC FEVER INCIDENCE IN DENMARK 1862 - 1962

Figure 2.2 Reported rheumatic fever incidence in Denmark, 1862–1962. Source: Public Health Board of Denmark, Copenhagen, Denmark. Notice how the decline in incidence started early in the century, before sulfonamides and pencillin, but accelerated after these agents became available

rate of these infections to the physical closeness between individuals (Figure 2.4).

Overcrowding may be one reason why the incidence of rheumatic fever seems to be increasing in many of the poorer developing countries. Industrialization has attracted many immigrants from rural areas seeking work in the cities, where they live in crowded slums. This population shift is reminiscent of that brought about by the industrial revolution in Western Europe during the last century, a time when the incidence of rheumatic fever was also high. In addition to crowding in the home, urbanization is accompanied by the increase in the number of children attending school and congregating in other communal activities outside the home. It is intriguing that in recent U.S. outbreaks most of the patients were relatively well off and lived in rural and suburban areas, but were crowded nevertheless[14].

Other components of the syndrome of poverty in the developing countries may also play a role. Availability and quality of medical care are part of the social environment; and since effective means for prevention exist, their availability is a significant "environmental factor." The marked acceleration in the decline of rheumatic fever in Western countries since the 1940s is attributable to medical intervention: greater availability of medical care and widespread use of antibiotics. It is also worth emphasizing that most of the original studies on prevention of rheumatic fever were carried out on indigent populations, and that the diligent administration of prophylactic drugs

15

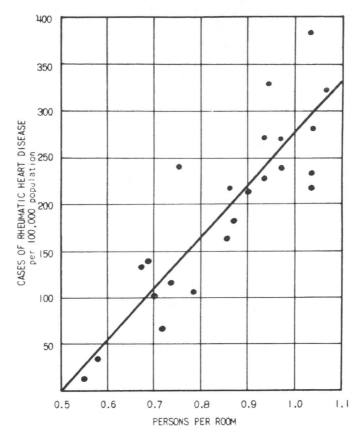

Figure 2.3 Relation of prevalence of rheumatic heart disease to crowding in the home. From Perry and Roberts (1937). *Br. Med. J.* (Suppl.), 28 August, p. 154

drastically reduced recurrences of rheumatic fever in these populations, even though their poor socioeconomic conditions remained unchanged.

Whether other manifestations of poverty directly influence rheumatic fever is a matter for conjecture. Nutrition affects immunity, and since immunologic mechanisms are involved in rheumatic fever it is reasonable to suspect that nutrition influences rheumatic fever as well, but whether it actually does so, we do not yet know.

References

1. Wannamaker, L. W. *et al.* (1951). Prophylaxis of acute rheumatic fever by treating the preceding streptococcal infection. *Am. J. Med.,* **10**, 673
2. Karoui, H. A. *et al.* (1982). Hemolytic streptococci and streptococcal antibodies in normal

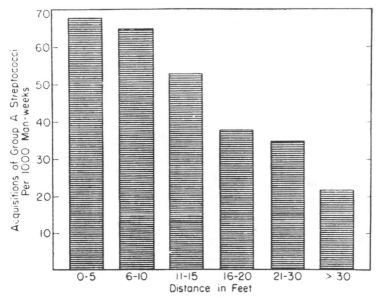

Figure 2.4 Acquisition rates (infection and colonization) for group A streptococci according to bed distance from the nearest carrier. From Wannamaker (1954), In McCarty, M. (ed.) *Streptococcal Infections.* New York: Columbia University Press

school children in Kuwait. *Am. J. Epidemiol.*, **116**, 709

3. Koshi, G. and Myers, R. M. (1971). Steptococcal disease in South India. *Indian J. Pathol. Bacteriol.*, **14**, 17
4. El-Kholy, A. M. *et al.* (1973). A three years' prospective study of steptococcal infections in a population of rural Egyptian school children. *J. Gen. Microbiol.*, **6**, 101
5. El-Batish, *et al.* (1985). Streptococcal pharyngitis in Kuwait: a pilot study in the community. *J. Kuwait Med. Assoc.*, **19**, 39
6. Rotta, J. (1974). Antistreptolysin O surveys in the populations of some Asian and African countries. In Haverkorn, M. (ed.), *Streptococcal Disease and the Community.* Amsterdam: Excerpta Medica
7. Rheumatic fever and rheumatic heart disease. Report of a WHO Study Group (1988). *WHO Technical Series* (in press)
8. Bisno, A. L. (1980). The concept of rheumatogenic and nephritogenic group A streptococci. In Read, S. E. and Zabriskie (eds.) *Steptococcal Diseases and the Immune Response.* New York: Academic Press
9. Majeed, A. M. *et al.* (1984). Acute rheumatic fever below the age of five years. *Ann. Trop. Paediatr.*, **4**, 37
10. Taranta, A. *et al.* (1959). Rheumatic fever in monozygotic and dizygotic twins. *Circulation*, **20**, 778
11. Spagnuolo, M. and Taranta, A. (1968). Rheumatic fever in siblings: similarity of its clinical manifestations. *N. Engl. J. Med.*, **278**, 183
12. Potarroyo, M. E. *et al.* (1979). Association of a B cell alloantigen with susceptibility to rheumatic fever. *Nature (London)*, **278**, 173
13. Zabriskie, J. B. *et al.* (1985). Rheumatic fever-associated B cell alloantigens as identified by

monoclonal antibodies. *Arthritis Rheum.*, **28**, 1047
14. Veasey, L. J. *et al.* (1987). Resurgence of acute rheumatic fever in the Intermountain Area of the U.S.A. *N. Engl. J. Med.*, **316**, 421–427
15. Woo, K. S. *et al.* (1983). The changing prevalence and pattern of acute rheumatic fever and rheumatic heart disease in Hong Kong (1968–1978). *Aust. N.Z. J. Med.*, **13**, 151

Chapter 3
Pathogenesis and pathology

Pathogenesis

A lot is known about the streptococcus, and a lot is known about rheumatic fever, but little is known about what connects the two: the chain of processes that must link the streptococcal infections in the throat to rheumatic fever itself – which starts *after* the pharyngitis has subsided and which only affects organs and tissues remote from the throat[1]. One thing is sure: the streptococci don't migrate from the throat to the heart or the joints, which are demonstrably sterile. Hence, rheumatic fever is considered a non-suppurative sequel of streptococcal infections; a *post-streptococcal* rather than a streptococcal disease.

The infection must be *in the throat*. The other common site for streptococcal infection is the skin[2], but while skin infections can lead to post-streptococcal glomerulonephritis, they don't lead to rheumatic fever (Figure 3.1). Streptococci that produce skin infections (streptococcal impetigo or pyoderma) usually are of different group A types from those that cause throat infection, but it is not clear whether this accounts for the difference in the capability to bring about rheumatic fever, or whether there are other differences which are crucial: anatomic, for instance. The ASO antibody response following a skin infection is much lower than after a throat infection, possibly due to inhibition of streptolysin O by skin lipids[3]; this difference could be the reason why streptococcal infections of the skin don't cause rheumatic fever, but there may be many other reasons as well.

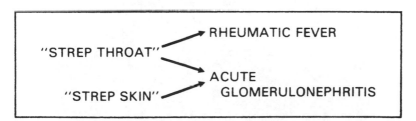

Figure 3.1 Relation of streptococcal infections of the throat and of the skin to post-streptococcal complications. Streptococcal infections of the throat ("strep throat") may lead to either rheumatic fever or acute glomerulonephritis, but streptococcal infections of the skin ("strep skin") may lead only to glomerulonephritis

19

As noted earlier, the streptococci must cause an *infection*, not just a coloniz-ation. Operationally, an infection is defined by the appearance of an anti-body response to any streptococcal antigen. To cause an infection the strep-tococci must first of all attach to the epithelial cells in the pharynx of the host, establish a beachhead there; and they do this by means of hair-like projec-tions called fimbriae, a sort of non-motile flagella. Virulent streptococci have fimbriae, avirulent ones don't[4] (Figure 3.2). In fact, one can digest away the fimbriae by delicately "shampooing" the streps with pepsin, and the result-ing "bald" streptococci will be incapable of infecting, i.e., will become avi-rulent, just like Samson became unable to fight after Delilah cut his hair[5].

What makes the fimbriae stick to the cells? If one pre-treats epithelial cells with lipoteichoic acid, a streptococcal cell component, the cells lose their capacity to get streptococci stuck to them (Figure 3.3). This strongly suggests that streptococci get attached to epithelial cells by means of lipoteichoic acid on the streptococcal side, and of a receptor for lipoteichoic acid on the epi-thelial cell side[6]. The M proteins, which are also located on the fimbriae, make it difficult for phagocytes to ingest the strep, thus further increasing virulence – unless the M proteins are neutralized by specific anti-M antibod-ies. That the attachment of lipoteichoic acid to human cells plays a role in the pathogenesis of rheumatic fever not only in permitting attachment, and

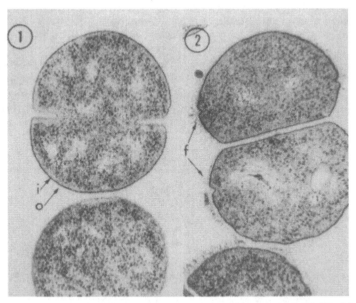

Figure 3.2 Streptococcal cells devoid of M protein (1) and endowed with it (2). The M protein is located in the fimbriae, visible only in (2) (f); i and o indicate the inner and outer layer of the cell wall. From ref. 4, with permission

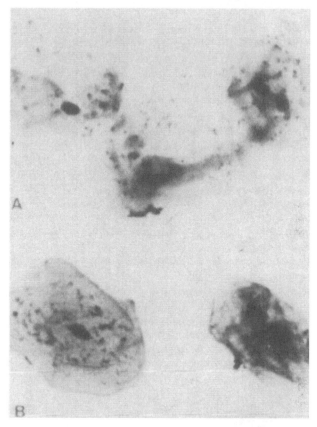

Figure 3.3 Inhibition of adherence of type 24 streptococci to buccal epithelial cells by lipoteichoic acid. (**A**) Control cells treated with phosphate-buffered saline. Notice the streptococci, mostly in short chains, adhering to the cells. (**B**) Epithelial cells pretreated with 1 mg/mL purified lipoteichoic acid. There are no streptococci adhering to the cells. From Ofek, I., Beachey, E. H., Jefferson, W. and Campbell, G. L. (1975). Cell membrane binding properties of group A streptococcal lipoteichoic acid. *J. Exp. Med.*, **141**, 990

therefore infection, but also in some additional and more direct way has been suggested[7], but remains uncertain.

Everybody agrees that "skin types" do not cause rheumatic fever (or, if you wish, are not "rheumatogenic") but what about the "throat types?" Conventional thinking holds that all types can induce rheumatic fever, as long as they can produce a pharyngitis[8]. But there have long been dissenting views, and they are gathering momentum.

Kuttner and Krumwiede, back in the 1930s, described an epidemic of streptococcal pharyngitis in a population of children convalescing from rheumatic fever – and therefore highly susceptible to recurrences[9]. Surprisingly, no recurrence ensued, while at the same time other epidemics of streptococcal pharyngitis caused by other types in the same population were dutifully followed by recurrences. To make the observation more striking, infection with type 4, which caused no recurrences, was accompanied by more symptoms than the infections with types 27 and C51, which did cause recurrences (Figure 3.4). This observation, and others like it collected by Stollerman[10] and Bisno[11] have kept alive the concept of *rheumatogenicity* – an elusive quality seemingly possessed by some, not all, pharyngeal types, or strains, of group A streptococci. The virtual disappearance of rheumatic fever in the 1970s[12] and its reappearance in the 1980s[13] certainly suggest some kind of change in the strep. (*Rheumatogenicity*, of course, is a concept analogous to that of *nephritogenicity*, the more widely accepted property of some streptococcal strains to cause acute glomerulonephritis. Although more accepted, nephritogenicity is still just that, a concept – still not endowed with a structural or chemical basis.)

A hyaluronic acid capsule, which further hinders phagocytosis and thus enhances virulence, is often found on rheumatogenic strains, especially in epidemic or near-epidemic streptococcal outbreaks. Such a capsule gives colonies on a blood agar plate a "juicy" mucoid appearance, which had not been seen for years but is reappearing now[14].

Although streptococci remain localized at the site of infection, the throat, their products diffuse out. Some of these products are cardiotoxic in experimental animals and could be the mediators of tissue damage in rheumatic fever, that is, they could damage the tissue by themselves, directly. The latent

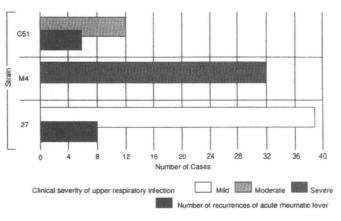

Figure 3.4 Rheumatogenicity or just chance? This graph, redrawn from the original data of Kuttner and Krumwiede[9] by Stollerman and Bisno, illustrates the striking difference in attack rate of rheumatic fever in three micro-epidemics of streptococcal pharyngitis in a highly susceptible population of children convalescing from rheumatic fever

period between the streptococcal infection and the onset of rheumatic fever is a stumbling block of this hypothesis, but not an insurmountable one: some toxins do act after a latent period (consider tetanus or diphtheritic myocarditis). Most toxins are antigenic, which is another stumbling block for the toxic hypothesis (because antibodies elicited by the toxins would be expected to protect against recurrences) but streptolysin S is not antigenic[15], which has made it an attractive candidate to some. Moreover, not all antibodies are neutralizing and not all antigen–antibody complexes are tight enough to preclude all biological actions of the antigen.

More popular than the toxin theory in recent decades (in fact, since the turn of the century) has been one version or another of an immunologic theory: allergy, hypersensitivity, and autoimmunity have been invoked, more notably and recently the last.

As the streptococcal products diffuse out of the pharyngeal epithelium they encounter, of course, lymphoid cells and stimulate antibody responses. Several streptococcal antigens happen to cross-react immunologically with human tissue antigens, though many of each set don't (Figure 3.5); as a result the immune response to streptococci may be blunted (as their antigens may be erroneously recognized as "self" by the lymphocytes) and whatever response is elicited may boomerang, in part, on the host (as the host's antigens may be mistaken as foreign). The latter "mistake" (autoimmunity) may be the mechanism whereby tissue damage in rheumatic fever comes about – especially rheumatic carditis, as the well-studied cross-reactions of streptococcal antigens with heart antigens suggest.

The number of reported cross-reactions has in fact led to an embarrassment of riches (Table 3.1), and in the absence of a laboratory model of rheumatic fever, which could put each cross-reaction to the acid test, it may be very difficult to unravel this tangle.

Why all these cross-reactions? Perhaps for the same reasons that a number of insects and "higher organisms" somehow resemble their background: so

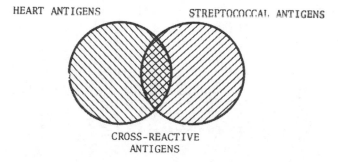

Figure 3.5 Schematic representation of the sets of human and streptococcal antigens and their interrelation

Table 3.1 Cross-reactions between streptococci and human tissues

Streptococcal component	Human component	Authors (year)
M-like protein in cell wall of some group A strains	Myocardium	Kaplan and Meyserian (1962)[16]
Glycoprotein of cell membrane	Glycoprotein of glomerular basement membrane	Markowitz and Lange (1964)[17]
Antigen of cell membrane	Histocompatibility antigen	Rapaport et al. (1966)[18]
Cell membranes of all group A strains	Myocardial sarcolemma?	Zabriskie and Freimer (1966)[19]
Type 1 streptococcal cells	Myocardial intercalated discs	Lyampert et al. (1966)[20]
Four distinct antigens in acid extracts of streptococcal cells	Four distinct myocardial antigens	Lyampert (1966)[21]
Group A polysaccharide	Glycoproteins of heart valves	Goldstein et al. (1967)[22]
Three distinct streptococcal antigens	Three distinct kidney antigens	Holm (1967)[23]
Streptococcal hyaluronic acid	Mammalian hyaluronic acid and protein polysaccharide	Sandson et al. (1968)[24]
Antigen of cell membrane	Neuronal cytoplasm of cordate and subthalamic nuclei	Husby et al. (1976)[25]

that they may "fade into it" and more easily escape predators – insectivorous birds in the case of butterflies, antibodies and phagocytes in the case of streptococci. Just as there is a visual mimicry among the butterflies of the Amazonian jungle, there may be a molecular mimicry, as it has been called, among the streptococci of the pharyngeal jungle. Both kinds of mimicry make sense in a world that lives by cheating, or at least survives by it.

Group A carbohydrate antibodies, which had been reported to cross-react with glycoprotein of the human heart valves[22] were reported to persist longer after rheumatic fever in patients with rheumatic heart disease than in those without it. Because of this observation, and because of the central role played by the heart valves in rheumatic carditis and in chronic rheumatic heart disease, group A carbohydrate antibodies and their cross-reaction have been the object of intensive pathogenetic speculation[26]. However, streptococcal infections of the skin, which are not rheumatogenic, elicit group A carbohydrate antibody just like infections of the throat, which are rheumatogenic[27]. And the difference in the rate of decrease of this antibody between patients with and without rheumatic heart disease could not be confirmed in a large series of patients in a blinded study done with a different method[28]. Finally, the level of group A antibody decreased after valvectomy but not after valvotomy[29], as if the group A antibodies persisted in patients with rheumatic heart disease because of continual self-immunization with the diseased valvular material still present in the heart. The prolonged persistence of group A carbohydrate antibodies would then be a consequence of valvular damage, rather than its cause, a chicken rather than an egg. The plot has surely thickened.

A number of other immunologic theories have been proposed over the years. Burnet suggested that lymphocytes affected by streptococcal products at the site of the infection activate "forbidden clones" with autoimmune activity[30]. A variant of this hypothesis holds that lymphocytes are transformed into blast cells *in vivo* by a streptococcal mitogen, which is immunologically non-specific but characteristic of group A, and the "transformed" lymphocytes might damage the host's tissues[31,32] in a manner analogous to the damage to syngeneic cells brought about *in vitro* by phytohemagglutinin-stimulated lymphocytes.

A mechanism akin to serum sickness or to the Arthus reaction has also been invoked: streptococcal antigens might persist in the body of the patient who will develop rheumatic fever and react with the corresponding antibodies, fix complement and damage tissues. Against this interpretation is the fact that the latent period of rheumatic fever does not get shorter on recurrences, while that of serum sickness characteristically does; in favor of it, however, is the recent finding of decreased complement components Clq, C3 and C4 in the synovial fluid of patients with rheumatic fever[33].

Considering the variety of manifestations of the rheumatic fever syndrome (some fleeting, others chronic; some exudative, others proliferative) it would not be surprising if more than one mechanism were involved.

Pathology

Carditis

In patients dying early in the disease, myocardial damage predominates. The heart muscle is flabby, edematous, pale, and mildly hypertrophic. The cardiac chambers are dilated. Endocarditis is almost invariably present: the valve leaflets have tiny transluscent nodules, or *verrucae*, on the edges, but are not grossly altered otherwise. The auricular endocardium may be thickened, especially in the left auricle, above the base of the posterior leaflet of the mitral valve ("McCallum patch"). The serofibrinous effusion of rheumatic pericarditis may also be found.

Microscopically, diffuse degeneration and swelling of muscle fibers may be apparent, along with fibrinoid degeneration of collagen. Perivascular foci of degeneration or necrosis may be surrounded by clusters of large mononuclear and giant multinuclear cells[34], largely of monocyte or macrophage lineage[35]. These clusters, known as Aschoff bodies or nodules, are considered specific for acute rheumatic fever; they may persist long after any other evidence of active disease but are often found later also (Figure 3.6). Immunofluorescent study reveals immunoglobulins and complement in cardiac myofibers, vessel walls[36], and pericardium[37]. Valvular lymphoid infiltrates contain a predominance of T-cells[38].

In patients who die in a later stage of the first attack, or with a recurrent

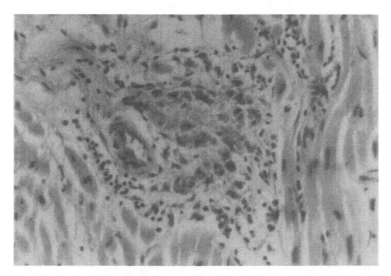

Figure 3.6 Typical myocardial Aschoff nodule in acute stage of rheumatic myocarditis. "Smudged" degenerated collagen, large mononuclear cells, and lymphocytes in characteristic perivascular location (× 270)

attack, the valve leaflets are retracted, thickened, and deformed. Their commissures may be fused, and the *chordae tendineae* may be retracted and fused. The valves may now share the responsibility for heart failure with the myocardial lesions.

However, most patients who die of rheumatic fever do so many years after the last acute attack. Deformed and sometimes calcified valves may themselves explain the congestive failure and death, although some Aschoff bodies, often partly fibrotic, or reduced to spindle-shaped or triangular scars, may still be found. The heart is regularly greatly enlarged because of both dilation and hypertrophy. In mitral stenosis, fibrin deposits in various stages of organization and fibrous replacement were found in 70% of cases. Some sections showed this process to have been recurrent. The repeated fibrin deposition followed by replacement with fibrous tissue leads to thickening of the cusps and narrowing of the orifice by a gradual "silting-up" process. Rheumatic pericarditis may lead to calcification, but not to constriction.

Arthritis

The articular and periarticular structures are swollen and edematous, but there is never erosion of the joint surfaces or pannus formation. The exudate is turbid but never purulent. At the outset it contains mostly polymorphonuclear leukocytes; later, mononuclear cells increase. Fibrin with enmeshed exudate cells may overlay the lining mesothelial membrane, which is proliferated and damaged. The deeper synovial layers may be infiltrated with polymorphonuclear leukocytes, small round cells, and multinucleated cells; the connective tissue fibers may be swollen and fibrinoid degeneration may be present.

Chorea

The few pathologic observations available, usually on patients who had died of carditis with concomitant chorea, have revealed arteritis, cellular degeneration, and occasional emboli and infarctions[35]. Such alterations involve areas scattered throughout the cortex, basal ganglia, substantia nigra, and cerebellum. The significance of these changes is unclear because of the lack of a consistent localization, and because similar findings have been reported in rheumatic fever without chorea.

Subcutaneous nodules

Subcutaneous nodules contain much fibrinoid material in strands with clear spaces between them. There is much edema and relatively few cells, most of which are fibroblasts or histiocytes with an occasional lymphocyte and a rare polymorph. Vascular "islands" are present, but there is no clear demarcation in concentric zones, and there is little palisading of cells. Fibrosis is not prominent[39].

27

References

1. Wannamaker, L. W. (1973). The chain that links the heart to the throat. T. Duckett Jones Memorial Lecture. *Circulation*, **48**, 9
2. Wannamaker, L. W. (1976). Differences between streptococcal infections of the throat and of the skin. *N. Engl. J. Med.*, **282**, 23, 78
3. Kaplan, E. L. and Wannamaker, L. W. (1974). Streptolysin O. Suppression of its antigenicity by lipids extracted from skin. *Proc. Soc. Exp. Biol. Med.*, **146**, 205
4. Swanson, J., Hsu, K. C. and Gotschlich, E. C. (1969). Electron microscopic studies on streptococci. I. M antigen. *J. Exp. Med.*, **130**, 10063
5. *The Holy Bible.* Judges, Chapter 16
6. Ofek, I. and Beachey, E. H. (1980). Bacterial adherence. *Adv. Intern. Med.*, **25**, 503
7. Williams, R. C. (1983). Rheumatic fever and the streptococcus. *Am. J. Med.*, **75**, 727
8. Rammelkamp, C. H., Jr (1955–56). *Harvey Lect., Series* **15**, 113
9. Kuttner, A. G. and Krumwiede, E. (1941). Observations on the effect of streptococcal upper respiratory infections on rheumatic children: a three-year study. *J. Clin. Invest.*, **20**, 273–287
10. Stollerman, G. H. (1969). Nephritogenic and rheumatogenic group A streptococci. *J. Infect. Dis.*, **120**, 258
11. Bisno, A. L. (1980). The concept of rheumatogenic and non-rheumatogenic group A streptococci. In Read, S. E. and Zabrirskie, J. B. (eds), *Streptococcal Diseases and the Immune Response.* New York: Academic Press, pp. 789–803
12. Gordis, L. (1985). The virtual disappearance of rheumatic fever in the United States: lessons in the rise and fall of disease. *Circulation*, **72**, 1155–1162
13. Veasy, L. G. *et al.* (1987). Resurgence of acute rheumatic fever in the intermountain area of the United States. *N. Engl. J. Med.*, **316**, 421–427
14. Kaplan, E. (1988). Personal communication
15. Stollerman, G. H. and Bernheimer, A. W. (1950). Inhibition of streptolysin S by the serum of patients with rheumatic fever and streptococcal pharyngitis. *J. Clin. Invest.*, **20**, 1147
16. Kaplan, M. H. and Meyeserian, M. (1962). An immunologic cross-reaction between group A streptococcal cells and human heart. *Lancet*, **1**, 706
17. Markowitz, A. S. and Lange, D. F. (1964). Streptococcal related glomerulonephritis. Isolation of soluble fractions from Type 12 streptococci. *J. Immunol.*, **92**, 565
18. Rappaport, F. T. *et al.* (1966). Transplantation activity of bacterial cells in different animal species. *Ann. N.Y. Acad. Sci.*, **129**, 102
19. Zabriskie, J. B. and Freimer, E. H. (1966). An immunologic relationship between group A streptococci and mammalian muscle. *J. Exp. Med.*, **124**, 661
20. Lyampert, I. M. *et al.* (1966). Mechanism of formation of antibodies to heart tissue in immunization with group A streptococci. *Folia Biol. (Praha)*, **12**, 108
21. Lyampert, I. M. (1966). Study on streptococcus group A antigens common with heart tissue elements. *Immunology*, **11**, 313
22. Goldstein, I. *et al.* (1967). Immunologic relationship between group A streptococcal polysaccharide and the structural glycoproteins of heart valves. *Nature*, **213**, 44
23. Holm, S. E. (1967). Precipitinogens in beta hemolytic streptococci and some related human kidney antigens. *Acta Pathol. Microbiol. Immunol. Scand.*, **70**, 79
24. Sandson, J. *et al.* (1968). Immunologic and chemical similarities between the streptococcus and human connective tissue. *Trans. Assoc. Am. Phys.*, **81**, 249
25. Husby, G. *et al.* (1976). Antibody reacting with cytoplasm of subthalamic and caudate nuclei neurons in chorea. *J. Exp. Med.*, **144**, 1094
26. Dudding, B. A. and Ayoub, E. M. (1968). Persistence of streptococcal group A antibody in patients with rheumatic valvular disease. *J. Exp. Med.*, **128**, 1081
27. Kaplan, E. L., *et al.* (1974). Fifth International Symposium on *Streptococcus pyogenes*, Amsterdam, Holland
28. Zimmerman, R. A., Auernheimer, A. H. and Taranta, A. (1971). Precipitating antibody

to Group A streptococcal polysaccharide in humans. *J. Immunol.*, **107**, 832–841

29. Ayoub, E. M., Taranta, A. and Bartley, T. D. (1974). Effect of valvular surgery on antibody to the group A streptococcal carbohydrate. *Circulation*, **50**, 144

30. Burnet, F. M. (1959). *The Clonal Selection Theory of Acquired Immunity.* Nashville, Tenn.: Vanderbilt University Press

31. Taranta, A., Cuppari, G. and Quagliata, F. (1969). Dissociation of hemolytic and lymphocyte-transforming activities of streptolysin S preparations. *J. Exp. Med.*, **129**, 605–622

32. Taranta, A. (1974). Lymphocyte mitogens of staphylococcal origin. *Ann. N.Y., Acad. Sci.*, **236**, 362

33. Svartman, M. *et al.* (1975). Immunoglobulins and complement components in synovial fluid of patients with acute rheumatic fever. *J. Clin. Invest.*, **56**, 111

34. Murphy, G. E. (1963). The characteristic rheumatic lesions of striated and of non-striated or smooth muscle cells of the heart. Genesis of the lesions known as Aschoff bodies and those myogenic components known as Aschoff cells or as Anitschkow cells or myocytes. *Medicine*, **42**, 73

35. Husby, G. *et al.* (1986). Immunofluorescence studies of florid rheumatic Aschoff lesions. *Arthritis Rheum.*, **2**, 207

36. Kaplan, M. H. *et al.* (1964). Presence of bound immunoglobulins and complement in myocardium in acute rheumatic fever. Association with cardiac failure. *N. Engl. J. Med.*, **271**, 637

37. Persellin, S. T., Ramirez, G. and Moatamed, F. (1982). Immunopathology of rheumatic pericarditis. *Arthritis Rheum.*, **25**, 1054

38. Raizada, V. *et al.* (1983). Tissue distribution of lymphocytes in rheumatic heart valves as defined by monoclonal anti-T cell antibodies. *Am. J. Med.*, **74**, 90

39. Benedek, T. G. (1984). Subcutaneous nodules and the differentiation of rheumatoid arthritis from rheumatic fever. *Semin. Arthritis Rheum.*, **4**, 305

Chapter 4
Clinical manifestations

The natural history of rheumatic fever may be said to start with the streptococcal pharyngitis that precedes it by an interval ("latent period") of 2 to 3
weeks (mean 18.6 days). The latent period of rheumatic fever is a little longer
than that of post-streptococcal glomerulonephritis, and is of the same length
in first attacks and in recurrences[1].

Mode of onset

If the only manifestation is carditis, the attack may have an insidious onset
with malaise and fatigue progressing to frank congestive heart failure, abdominal pain due to acute liver distension, and dyspnea. Peripheral edema and
pulmonary rales are late manifestations in children. If pericarditis is also present, precordial pain may appear acutely. Cardiac tamponade may ensue,
with pulsus paradoxicus and even syncope due to decreased venous return
to the right heart. Patients whose main manifestation is carditis often have
arthralgias, which are often ignored or neglected and interpreted as part of
a rheumatic fever attack only in retrospect.

When arthritis is part of the picture, the onset is characteristically acute.
With chorea the onset may appear to be acute, but there may have been sub-
tle behavior changes before that, which can be interpreted as part of chorea
only in retrospect.

Carditis

This is the most serious manifestation of rheumatic fever because it is the only
one that can cause death during the acute attack, or that may leave behind
structural abnormalities which can entail residual disability and late mortality. Its severity may vary from a fulminating, fatal course to an entirely
asymptomatic one. In the latter case carditis is often diagnosed on the basis
of physical signs only in a patient who comes to medical attention because of
non-cardiac symptoms, such as joint pains or chorea. However, whenever
medical facilities are scarce, carditis is often diagnosed in patients coming to
medical attention because of symptoms more serious than transient pain in
the joints or involuntary movements, i.e., cardiac symptoms: shortness of
breath, dependent edema, right upper quadrant pain (caused by acute distension of the liver), or precordial pain caused by pericarditis. In either case

the physical signs are mostly found on *auscultation:* organic heart murmurs and sometimes pericardial friction rubs. It is a good custom, however, to *palpate* the heart also, as vibrations of low frequency may be picked up in this way, as long as they have the necessary intensity. Even inspection is valuable, as it may reveal a precordial bulge in children with severe cardiomegaly, venous distension, and arterial collapse during diastole in aortic regurgitation.

If carditis does not appear within the first 2 or 3 weeks of the attack, it seldom appears later.

Murmurs

The most commonly heard murmur during acute rheumatic fever is an organic systolic murmur at the apex, which indicates mitral regurgitation. It is long, and usually lasts the whole of systole (pansystolic or holosystolic murmur); its loudness is at least grade 2 on a scale of 6, but usually grade 3/6 or more; its pitch tends to be high and its character blowing. Because of its loudness the murmur can be heard also in the axilla. Mitral regurgitation murmurs are not obliterated by inspiration or postural changes.

Another murmur that is often heard in association with mitral regurgitation is an apical mid-diastolic murmur (Carey Coombs murmur), which starts with the third heart sound and ends distinctly before the first heart sound. It should be differentiated from the murmur of established mitral stenosis (which is rumbling in character, is often preceded by the opening "snap" of the mitral valve, and, in the presence of a sinus rhythm, is accentuated in presystole – due to accelerated blood flow produced by the "atrial kick", i.e., the increase in flow due to the atrial contraction). Whereas the murmur of established mitral stenosis is due to actual narrowing of the valve orifice, the Carey Coombs murmur appears to be due to "relative" stenosis of the mitral valve in relation to the dilated ventricular chamber, often combined with a large inflow of blood into the left ventricle early in diastole. In addition to these acutely developing murmurs, a murmur of mitral stenosis may also be found during the acute attack (especially in developing countries where a first attack may be more frequently missed); it indicates that the patient has had a previous attack of rheumatic fever (even if the previous attack was forgotten or never diagnosed).

Less frequent than the apical murmurs is the diastolic murmur indicative of aortic regurgitation. This is a high-pitched, blowing murmur of "decrescendo" intensity. It is usually heard best along the left sternal border over the third or second interspace. It may be short and faint and then difficult to hear[2]. Soft systolic murmurs are frequently heard at the base of the heart in normal subjects, but a loud "diamond-shaped" or crescendo–decrescendo murmur accompanied by a thrill and by a decreased second heart sound indicates aortic stenosis. It may be heard during the acute attack, especially in developing countries, and then indicates, just like mitral stenosis, that the patient has had at least one previous rheumatic attack, since it takes years to develop aortic stenosis.

Pericardial friction rubs

These are scratchy, crunchy, crackling or leathery sounds that can sometimes be altered by varying the pressure of the stethoscope against the chest wall. They are usually found in more than one phase of the cardiac cycle (systole as well as diastole), and may sometimes vary with the phase of respiration (pleuropericardial rubs). Auscultatory findings suggestive of pericarditis may be objects of dispute: someone hears them, someone else doesn't. EKG, chest X-ray, phonocardiography, and echocardiography most of all may help in making an "objective" diagnosis.

Other auscultatory findings

In patients with carditis, tachycardia is disproportionate to the degree of fever and is present even during sleep ("sleeping tachycardia"), unlike emotional tachycardia. It often persists even after the temperature returns to normal.

Gallop rhythm is usually protodiastolic, resulting from accentuation of the third heart sound. Less frequently it is presystolic, resulting from accentuation of the usually inaudible fourth heart sound, or is a combination of the two ("summation" gallop).

The first heart sound often becomes indistinct, "impure," or "mushy" due to a first-degree A-V block which, by delaying ventricular contraction, allows the mitral leaflets to float back toward the atria before systole. The heart sounds may acquire a fetal or "tic-tac" quality. Both heart sounds may become indistinct whenever a large amount of fluid accumulates in the pericardium.

Silent carditis

Up to 50% of patients with the physical findings of rheumatic heart disease deny any history of rheumatic fever attacks. It is assumed that these patients had an attack of rheumatic fever involving the heart, but without pericarditis or congestive failure, and with neither polyarthritis nor chorea (and therefore asymptomatic). In such cases, because of the absence of symptoms, the physician will not be consulted and the carditis will be missed. In other cases symptoms may be vague, or the patient may be stoic, or a doctor just not available and the final result may be the same. Thus the disease may run its early course unrecognized: an episode of "silent carditis." This situation may be especially common wherever medical care is scarce.

Another possibility, however, is that the heart disease in some of these patients (with physical findings indicative of rheumatic heart disease but no history of a rheumatic attack) might have an etiology other than rheumatic fever, such as viral or congenital. Mitral regurgitation is the most common lesion of rheumatic heart disease, but when unaccompanied by mitral stenosis or aortic valve disease it may be due to other forms of valve disease, such as mitral valve prolapse. Aortic valve disease may be due to other causes such as congenital bicuspid valve. In the absence of mitral valve involvement, aortic valve disease is rarely rheumatic, but rheumatic mitral valve involvement may have been present earlier, and may have healed, leaving behind a seemingly isolated aortic involvement[3,4]. It thus appears that patients with valvular heart disease are a mixed bag: some have had an attack of silent rheumatic carditis, while others have heart disease of a different etiology.

Joint involvement

This ranges from arthralgia, i.e., joint pain without objective signs of inflammation, to arthritis, i.e., joint pains with objective signs of inflammation (heat, redness, swelling or tenderness to touch or definite limitation of motion). Objective signs, of course, depend for their detection on the skill and diligence of the examiner (hence the quip: "Arthralgia is arthritis minus a good physical examination"). Arthralgia and arthritis in rheumatic fever usually affect more than one joint, and are then called polyarthralgia and polyarthritis.

In most series of patients, arthritis is the most common manifestation of rheumatic fever but is not, of course, the most serious. As Lasègue so memorably put it, "*rheumatic fever licks the joints but bites the heart,*" and the polyarthritis or rheumatic fever has yet to recover from this "put-down." Yet this distinctive migratory polyarthritis has been important in characterizing the disease, and is useful in drawing attention to the patient and making the diagnosis easier. (Think of the diagnostic puzzle of "isolated carditis"!). In this sense, indeed, the arthritis of rheumatic fever is "the diagnostician's friend."

Joint involvement occurs early in the rheumatic attack. Usually it is exquisitely painful: the pain is more marked than the swelling. One seldom sees definitely swollen joints that are only slightly tender (as they may be in juvenile rheumatoid arthritis).

The arthritis of rheumatic fever affects several joints one after the other, and each for only a few days to a week. The term "migrating" or "migratory" is often used to describe the polyarthritis of rheumatic fever, but this does not mean that the inflammation disappears in one joint before it appears in another. Rather, the individual joint involvements overlap in time (Figure 4.1). The term "flitting" has also been used, but it gives a misleading impression of excessive speed in migration, which in fact is more a matter of days than of hours.

Arthritis often affects the legs first and then spreads to the arms. The knees

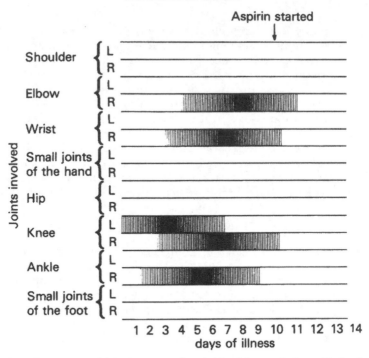

Figure 4.1 Time course of the migratory polyarthritis of rheumatic fever. Notice that, even in the absence of treatment, the involvement of each joint is short-lived, but the cumulative involvement of all joints is less so, and that arthritis rapidly responds to aspirin

are most frequently affected (75%) followed by the ankles (50%), elbows, wrists, hips, and small joints of the feet (each 12–15%), shoulders and small joints of the hand (7–8%). The involvement of other joints is rare: cervical spine, lumbosacral, sternoclavicular, and temporomandibular; and so is isolated involvement of small joints of the hands (i.e., without any other joint)[5]. Radiologic examination of the joints is negative, except for effusion. Most patients with arthritis are usually treated with aspirin or other drugs, so that the arthritis subsides quickly in the joint(s) already affected and does not migrate to new joints.

Arthritis may be just a lick to a joint, as Lasèque put it, but is nothing to dismiss or slight. It must be paid attention to, not only when it's severe and may really distress the patient, but also when it's not and may still give you the diagnosis. Before rushing to the laboratory for another mindless "collagen screen," let's examine the patient carefully, question him or her leisurely and repeatedly, and describe the symptoms and signs with appropriate attention to detail. To tell a rheumatologist, or just a plain good doctor, that the patient had "arthritis" and let it go at that, is like telling a Frenchman that one ate "cheese" without saying which of the 478 varieties.

Jaccoud's arthritis

Jaccoud's arthritis is also called, more descriptively, chronic post-rheumatic fever arthropathy. It is a rare, indolent, slowly progressive process that deforms the fingers and sometimes the toes[6]. The deformity consists of ulnar deviation of the fingers, flexion of the metacarpophalangeal joints, and hyperextension of the proximal interphalangeal joints, just as it occurs in rheumatoid arthritis, but without the inflammatory signs of the latter. The ulnar deviation occurs mostly in the fourth and fifth digits and is correctable at first, but later may become fixed. Rheumatoid factor is absent; the erythrocyte sedimentation is normal.

In classic cases, Jaccoud's arthropathy appears after multiple, prolonged, and severe attacks of rheumatic fever. It is thought to be the end result of the repeated inflammation of the fibrous articular capsules in the small joints of the hand (which are not frequently affected in rheumatic fever, and almost never by themselves alone), perhaps depending on individual predisposition. Patients with systemic lupus erythematosus (SLE) may develop a similar arthropathy[7], and some patients develop it without either SLE or rheumatic fever[8]. The prognosis of Jaccoud's arthropathy is good. Patients, alarmed by the deformity, may fear that it will extend to joints in other parts of the body, but this does not happen.

Chorea

Sydenham's chorea, chorea minor, or "St Vitus' dance" is a neurological disorder consisting of involuntary movements, muscular weakness, and emotional disturbances. The movements are abrupt and purposeless, not rhythmic or repetitive. They disappear during sleep, but may occur at rest and may interfere with voluntary activity. The movements can be suppressed by the will of the patient, but only for a short time. They may affect all voluntary muscles, but the involvement of the hands and face is usually the most obvious. Peculiar facial expressions or grimaces and inappropriate smiling are common (Figure 4.2). Handwriting usually becomes clumsy (a convenient way of following and documenting the patient's course is to ask her to write or to draw a spiral on a sheet of paper every day). Speech is often slurred. The movements are commonly more marked on one side, and are occasionally completely unilateral (hemichorea).

The muscular weakness is best revealed by asking the patient to squeeze the examiner's hands. The examiner will feel that the pressure of the patient's grip increases and decreases continuously and capriciously: "relapsing grip" or "milking sign."

The emotional changes manifest themselves in outbursts of inappropriate behavior, including crying and restlessness. The patients are frustrated at being unable to control their body, to perform the activities of daily living

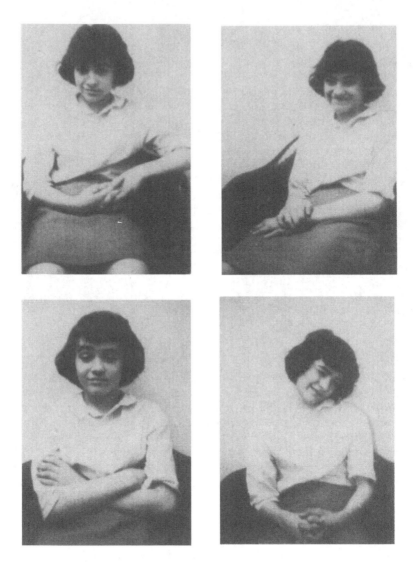

Figure 4.2 Inappropriate smiles, bizarre expressions or grimaces in a child with Sydenham's chorea

competently, and at being made fun of by children and scolded by adults. In exceptional cases the psychological manifestations may be quite severe, and result in transient psychosis ("chorea insaniens").

The neurological examination does not reveal sensory losses or pyramidal

36

tract involvement. There may be diffuse hypotonia. The choreic movements can be brought out in doubtful cases by asking the patient to stretch her hands in front of her, to stretch her fingers out, to close her eyes and to stick her tongue out, one movement on top of the other. By the time the tongue is stuck out, the fingers wiggle, or the eyelids flutter. When the arms are projected straight forward there is flexion of the wrist, hyperextension of the metacarpophalangeal joints, straightening of the fingers, and abduction of the thumb ("spooning" or "dishing" of the hands) (Figure 4.3). When the patient is asked to raise her arms above her head, she may also pronate one or both hands (pronator sign) (Figure 4.4).

Chorea may follow streptococcal infections after a latent period that is longer, on the average, than the latent period of other rheumatic manifestations[9]. Some patients with chorea have no other symptoms[10], but other patients develop chorea weeks or months after arthritis. In both cases, examination of the heart may reveal murmurs (Figure 4.5).

The incidence of chorea among rheumatic attacks has varied widely and seemed to be decreasing, but in the recent Utah epidemic it was 31%[11]. Chorea is unusual after puberty, and does not occur in adults, with the exception of rare cases during pregnancy ("chorea gravidarum"). Finally, it is the only manifestation with a marked sex preference. Chorea is twice as frequent in girls as in boys; after puberty this sex preference increases[12].

Subcutaneous nodules

Rheumatic subcutaneous nodules usually appear only after the first few weeks of illness and most of the time only in patients with carditis. They are firm and painless. The overlying skin is not inflamed, and almost invariably can be moved over them. The nodules are approximately round, and their

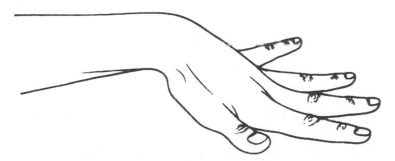

Figure 4.3 "Spooning" or "dishing" of the hands (flexion of the wrist and hyperextension of the metacarpophalangeal joints and of the interphalangeal joints) which is characteristically observed in children with Sydenham's chorea when they are asked to put their hands in front of them

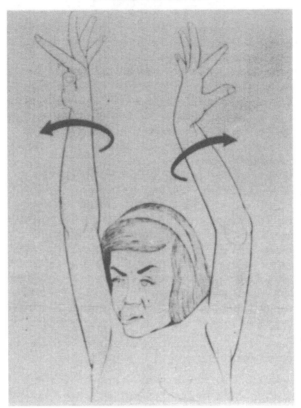

Figure 4.4 "Pronator sign" in a patient with Sydenham's chorea. When the child is asked to raise the arms above the head, the hands involuntarily rotate into pronation

diameter varies from a few millimeters to 1 or 2 cm. They last 1 or more weeks, rarely more than a month. They are usually smaller and last for a shorter time than the nodules of rheumatoid arthritis (Figure 4.6). The frequency of their appearance, or rather of their detection, varies widely from 34%[13] to 2%[14]. Subcutaneous nodules are very rare in adults with rheumatic fever, while in rheumatoid arthritis they are common in adults and rare in children.

Erythema marginatum

Erythema marginatum usually occurs in the early stage of the rheumatic fever attack. It often persists or returns later, even after all other manifestations of the disease have disappeared; or it may occasionally appear for the first time (or be noticed for the first time) later in the course of the illness, or even during convalesence. Like subcutaneous nodules, erythema marginatum usually occurs only in patients with carditis. It is a transient, non-pruritic

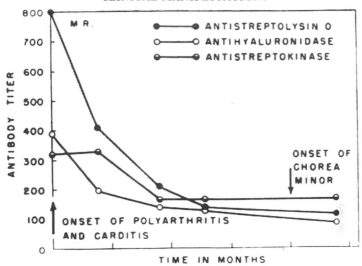

Figure 4.5 Chorea appearing 4 months after the onset of polyarthritis and carditis. Intercurrent streptococcal infections were ruled out by the falling titers of three streptococcal antibodies (from ref. 9)

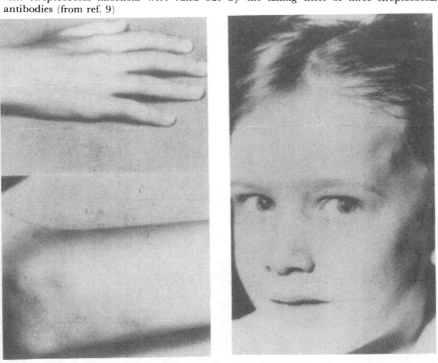

Figure 4.6 Subcutaneous nodules in a child with rheumatic fever. Notice that some of them are difficult to see: often they can be more easily felt than seen

39

skin rash, pink or faintly red, usually affecting the trunk, sometimes the proximal parts of the limbs, but never the face (Figure 4.7). It consists of a variable number of erythematous patches of 1–3 cm diameter, which may be slightly raised. Each lesion extends centrifugally while the skin in the center clears, so that the outer margins are sharp while the inner margin is soft and blurry. The margin of the lesion is usually continuous, making a ring; hence the other name, "erythema annulare." The individual lesions may appear and disappear in a few hours, usually to return and disappear again. A hot bath or shower may make them more evident, or even bring them out for the first time.

Erythema marginatum is not considered a common manifestation, perhaps because it's evanescent and we don't look at our patients often enough. The reported incidence has varied from $13\%^{15}$ to $2\%^{14}$. It may be difficult to see in dark-skinned patients, and is particularly rare in adults.

Other manifestations

Fever

Fever is almost always present at the onset of rheumatic polyarthritis; it is often present in isolated carditis but not in isolated chorea. It is a remittent type of fever, without the wide diurnal variations typical of juvenile

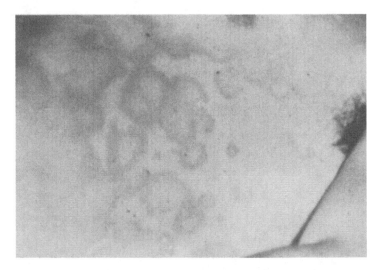

Figure 4.7 Erythema marginatum: notice the sharp outer edge of each individual lesion, the soft inner edge, and the confluence of lesions resulting in a festooned or circinate pattern (from the teaching slide collection of the American Rheumatism Association)

rheumatoid arthritis systemic onset type. In rheumatic fever the temperature rarely exceeds 39°C and returns to normal or near-normal in 2 or 3 weeks in most cases, even without treatment.

Abdominal pain and other unusual manifestations

Abdominal pain may occur in rheumatic fever with congestive heart failure, due to distension of the liver. It may also occur in rare cases without heart failure, and before any other specific manifestation of the disease. In these cases the pain may be severe in the periumbilical area. It occasionally leads to an unnecessary appendectomy.

Anorexia, nausea, and vomiting often occur, but mostly due to congestive heart failure, or salicylate toxicity. Severe epistaxis may occur. Fatigue is a vague and infrequent symptom, unless heart failure is present.

Other clinical manifestations, which are rarely seen nowadays in the West, are erythema nodosum, pleurisy, and "rheumatic pneumonia." It must be noted that congestive heart failure may be misdiagnosed as pleurisy or pneumonia, because of pleural effusion or pulmonary congestion, respectively. Therefore, "rheumatic pneumonia," if it exists at all, is both rare and difficult to diagnose.

Duration of the rheumatic attack

Duration as a whole (as opposed to the duration of each manifestation) varies according to the criterion used to determine it, and to the clinical manifestations present. It is the shortest in attacks characterized by arthritis alone; it is longer in the presence of chorea and longest in the presence of carditis. It is generally shorter if the end-point is disappearance of acute clinical manifestations, and longer if the end-point is return to normal of the sedimentation rate, although in some cases certain major clinical manifestations (chorea, and occasionally erythema marginatum and nodules) may persist or even appear for the first time after the acute phase reactants have returned to normal.

The duration of an initial attack of rheumatic fever ranges from less than 6 weeks (in one-third of cases) to 3 months. However, in patients with severe carditis, the active rheumatic process may continue for 6 months or more. These patients have "chronic" rheumatic fever. In Western countries this occurs in a small proportion of cases (3% or less). The majority of patients with protracted rheumatic fever have had multiple attacks. In countries where severe carditis and recurrences are common, the frequency of chronic rheumatic fever is probably higher.

The rheumatic fever process is considered active when any of the following is present: arthritis, new organic murmurs, enlarging heart size, a sleeping pulse of greater than 100/min, chorea, erythema marginatum, or subcutaneous nodules. Congestive heart failure in the absence of long-standing severe valvular disease is also a sign of active carditis. Chronic rheumatic carditis may be intractable and lead to death after many months or even several years. Persistence of an elevated sedimentation rate (ESR) for more than 6 months should not be considered a sign of rheumatic activity if no clinical signs are present.

Rheumatic fever in the adult

Streptococcal sore throats become less frequent as one becomes adult, and even the mean titer of streptococcal antibodies goes down. It's not surprising then that rheumatic fever is less common in adults, and is especially rare in the middle-aged and the elderly. This trend applies to recurrences as well as to first attacks, but because of the tendency of rheumatic fever to recur, a clinician will be less surprised by its reappearance than by its onset *de novo* in someone past adolescence. Environmental conditions may override this trend, however: during a war, or whenever large groups of young adults are crowded together, rheumatic fever, even epidemic rheumatic fever, may erupt.

More surprising, and in fact still unexplained, is the change in pattern of rheumatic fever manifestations. As the child matures, the susceptibility of its heart to rheumatic carditis, at least to significant valvular and myocardial involvement, decreases; and adults seldom if ever develop rheumatic carditis, unless they already had it in a previous attack. PR prolongation and other EKG changes do occur, however. Chorea is even more rigidly limited to children, though the susceptibility to it lingers a bit longer in girls than in boys and (very rarely) reappears in pregnancy ("chorea gravidarum"). Subcutaneous nodules and erythema marginatum, which are seen only in patients with carditis, are not seen in adults either.

What is left, then, is arthritis, which, by default, fills the statistics of rheumatic fever in the adult[16]. It also seems to be a bit more severe and more extensive, and to last longer than in children; but these differences are slight, and may even be due to a bias of selection (in the absence of carditis, mild cases of arthritis may escape hospitalization or even medical attention altogether).

References

1. Rammelkamp, C. H. Jr and Stolzer, B. L. (1961–62). The latent period before the onset of acute rheumatic fever. *Yale J. Biol. Med.*, **34**, 386
2. Feinstein, A. R. and DiMassa, R. (1960). The unheard diastolic murmur or aortic regurgitation. *N. Engl. J. Med.*, **262**, 533

3. Roberts, W. C. (1970). Anatomically isolated aortic valvular disease. The case against its being of rheumatic etiology. *Am. J. Med.*, **49**, 151
4. Spagnuolo, M. *et al.* (1971). Natural history of rheumatic aortic regurgitation. *Circulation*, **44**, 368
5. Feinstein, A. R. and Spagnuolo, M. (1962). The patterns of acute rheumatic fever revisited. *Medicine*, **41**, 279
6. Bittl, J. A. and Perloff, J. K. (1983). Chronic post-rheumatic fever arthropathy of Jaccoud. *Am. Heart J.*, **105**, 515
7. Bywaters, E. G. L. (1975). Jaccoud's syndrome: a sequel to the joint involvement of systemic lupus erythematosus. *Clin. Rheum. Dis.*, **1**, 125
8. Ignacak, T. *et al.* (1975). Jaccoud arthritis. *Arch. Intern. Med.*, **35**, 577
9. Taranta, A. and Stollerman, G. H. (1956). The relation of Sydenham's chorea to preceding streptococcal infections. *Am. J. Med.*, **20**, 170
10. Taranta, A. (1959). Relation of isolated recurrences of Sydenham's chorea to preceding streptococcal infections. *N. Engl. J. Med.*, **260**, 1204
11. Veasy, L. G. *et al.* (1987). Resurgence of acute rheumatic fever in the Intermountain Area of the United States. *N. Engl. J. Med.*, **316**, 421–427
12. Aron, A. M., Freeman, J. M. and Carter, S. (1965). The natural history of Sydenham's chorea. Review of the literature and long-term evaluation with emphasis on cardiac sequelae. *Am. J. Med.*, **38**, 83
13. Bywaters, E. G. L. and Thomas, G. T. (1961). Bed rest, salicylates and steroids in rheumatic fever. *Br. Med. J.*, **1**, 1628
14. Sanyal, S. K. *et al.* (1974). Sequelae of the initial attack of rheumatic fever in children from North India. *Circulation*, **49**, 7
15. United Kingdom and United States Joint report (1955). The natural history of rheumatic fever and rheumatic heart disease. Ten-year report of a cooperative clinical trial. *Circulation*, **11**, 343
16. Barnert, A. L., Jerry, E. E. and Persellin, R. H. (1975). Acute rheumatic fever in adults. *J. Am. Med. Assoc.*, **232**, 925

Chapter 5
Laboratory manifestations

There are three main kinds of laboratory tests that are useful for the diagnosis and management of rheumatic fever: tests to detect a preceding streptococcal infection, tests to measure "systemic inflammation," and tests to gauge the involvement of the heart. Additional studies may be useful to exclude other diseases which can mimic rheumatic fever; these are discussed under differential diagnosis.

Evidence of a recent streptococcal infection

Streptococcal antibody determinations are the only reliable test to detect a preceding streptococcal infection. They are usually elevated by the time the rheumatic fever attack starts. About 80% of patients with acute rheumatic fever have an elevated anti-streptolysin O (ASO) level, and the remaining 20% have a rise in one or the other streptococcal antibody tests (Figure 5.1)[1]. A throat culture is not very helpful because by the time signs and symptoms of acute rheumatic fever appear, the culture is usually negative, especially if antibiotics have been given for the preceding upper respiratory infection.

Generally, streptococcal antibody levels begin to decline within a month or two, so that they are helpful only if the patient is observed early in the

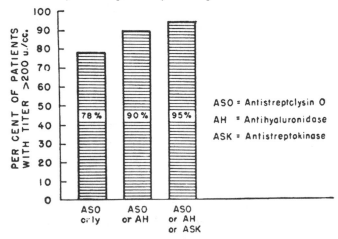

Figure 5.1 Streptococcal antibody titers in 88 patients studied within 2 months of onset of acute rheumatic fever (from Stollerman *et al.* (1956). *Am. J. Med.,* **20**, 163)

44

course of the acute rheumatic attack. Thus, in patients with insidious rheumatic carditis that is discovered several months after onset, streptococcal antibodies will usually have returned to normal levels. This is also true in patients with Sydenham's chorea, because this manifestation may sometimes appear several months after the streptococcal infection[2].

Occasionally, both a high and a low streptococcal antibody titer may mislead. A moderately high titer, for instance, may be the remnant of a much higher titer of many months before – and thus *not* be evidence of a *recent* infection. Conversely, a "low titer" may be high in relation to an even lower baseline level – and thus not be reliable evidence *against* a recent infection. Much more reliable than absolute titers are *changes* in titer: the comparison of acute and convalescent sera, just like in viral infections. Increases are most valuable, if they can be caught in time; but decreases in titer also are more reliable indicators of recent infection than a single determination. Because antibody determinations are serological tests of limited precision and reproducibility, it's best to store the "acute serum" in a freezer and test it side by side with a "convalescent" serum, thus cutting down on any unwitting variation in the conditions of the test from day to day. Two weeks' interval between the two serum samples is usually appropriate.

The ASO test is the best-standardized and the most frequently determined antibody test. The titers vary with intensity of exposure to streptococcal infections, which is influenced by age and geographic area. Titers up to 200 are common in healthy school-age children in the cities of north temperate zones so that only levels of 333 units or higher are considered abnormal[3]. In older subjects "normal" titers are lower. Ideally, each area should determine the range of titers in healthy individuals in different age groups to provide local standards.

In recent years a rapid hemagglutination test has been introduced for the detection of antibodies against a mixture of streptococcal antigens ("streptozyme"), but there have been problems with its reproducibility, and it is not recommended by the World Health Organization[4].

While streptococcal antibody tests are very useful to support the diagnosis of rheumatic fever, and under certain circumstances can rule out this diagnosis, the finding of increased antibodies does not "prove" the diagnosis, because streptococcal infections are so much more common than rheumatic fever. Furthermore, streptococcal antibodies are not a measure of the severity of the attack, nor of the persistence of rheumatic activity. Thus, there is no reason to repeat streptococal antibody tests after the diagnosis of acute rheumatic fever has been clearly established.

Evidence of systemic inflammation

Acute rheumatic fever is an inflammatory disease and a number of tests are available to measure presence and degree of a systemic inflammatory state.

The erythrocyte sedimentation rate (ESR) and the C-reactive protein test (CRP) are the best-known and most commonly used. Neither of these tests is specific for rheumatic fever, but they are very sensitive. For example, in patients with complaints suggestive of *acute* rheumatic fever, a normal ESR or negative CRP makes it highly unlikely that the symptoms are rheumatic. On the other hand, if these tests are abnormal, such patients should be re-examined at close intervals for other evidence of disease.

Both the ESR and CRP reflect the magnitude of the inflammatory process ("rheumatic activity"), and are useful to find out if the inflammatory process is still going on after the symptoms and signs have subsided. The CRP test is somewhat better for this purpose since it is regularly negative in healthy subjects, while the ESR has a gray zone between normal and abnormal.

Laboratory evidence of heart involvement

Radiography of the heart, echocardiography, and electrocardiography are the methods most often used to detect heart involvement, yet they are not universally labeled "laboratory", as they have all moved close to the bedside. Enlargement of the heart, pericardial effusion, and valve deformities are all to be looked for – and a detailed discussion of them is beyond the limits we have imposed on this book.

Electrocardiographic findings are of interest, although they lend themselves to misinterpretation. Prolongation of the P–R interval occurs in 28–40% of the patients; i.e., much more frequently than in other febrile illnesses, and is therefore *useful in the diagnosis of rheumatic fever*[5]. This usefulness is recognized and codified in the Jones criteria, which list P–R prolongation as a *minor criterion*; but P–R prolongation does not correlate with the presence or future development of valvular involvement, as detected by the auscultation of the heart[6]; the P–R interval therefore has no diagnostic value for carditis as classically defined, nor prognostic value. Other arrhythmias may include second degree A-V block, A-V dissociation, and even complete A-V block.

Doppler ultrasonography has proven to be useful to identify evidence of valvular involvement in patients with negative cardiac findings on physical examination. In a study of a recent outbreak in the United States involving 74 patients with an initial attack of acute rheumatic fever, 67 (91%) had cardiac involvement and, of these, mitral regurgitation was found by Doppler in 19 patients in whom no murmur could be detected[7]. Because Doppler evidence of mild mitral regurgitation can be found in normal people, further studies using this technique are needed[8]. It could prove to be extremely useful for identifying valvular involvement in patients with single clinical manifestations such as polyarthritis or chorea.

References

1. Stollerman, G. H. *et al.* (1956). Relationship of immune response to group A streptococci to the course of acute chronic and recurrent rheumatic fever. *Am. J. Med.*, **20**, 163
2. Taranta, A. and Stollerman, G. H. (1956). The relationship of Sydenham's chorea to infection with group A streptococci. *Am. J. Med.*, **20**, 170
3. American Heart Association (1984). Jones criteria (revised) for guidance in the diagnosis of rheumatic fever. *Circulation*, **69**, 204A
4. World Health Organization (1986). Evaluation of the streptozyme test for streptococcal antibodies. *Bull. WHO*, **64**, 504
5. Mirowski, M., Rosenstein, B. J. and Markowitz, M. (1964). A comparison of atrioventricular conduction in normal children and in patients with rheumatic fever, glomerulonephritis, and acute febrile illnesses. A quantitative study with determination of the P–R index. *Pediatrics*, **33**, 334
6. Feinstein, A. R. and Spagnuolo, M. (1959). Prognostic significance of valvular involvement in acute rheumatic fever. *N. Engl. J. Med.*, **260**, 1001
7. Veasey, L. J. *et al.* (1987). Resurgence of acute rheumatic fever in the Intermountain Area of the U.S.A. *N. Engl. J. Med.*, **316**, 421–427
8. Kostucki, W. *et al.* (1986). Pulsed Doppler regurgitant flow patterns of normal valves. *Am. J. Cardiol.*, **58**, 309

Chapter 6
Diagnosis

Unlike pneumococcal pneumonia, which invariably affects the lungs, rheumatic fever has no obligate target organ. It may affect a number of organs and tissues, singly or in combination. No single manifestation, with the exception of "pure" Sydenham's chorea (after other causes of choreiform movement have been excluded), or laboratory test is characteristic enough to be diagnostic, and therefore the diagnosis is based on appropriate combinations of them. The greater the number of manifestations, the firmer the diagnosis. Because the prognosis varies according to the clinical manifestation, the diagnosis should be qualified by mention of the clinical manifestation, e.g., rheumatic fever with polyarthritis only.

Jones criteria

In 1944 Dr T. Duckett Jones proposed diagnostic criteria based on combinations of clinical manifestations and laboratory findings according to their diagnostic usefulness[1]. Clinical signs that are most useful are designated *major manifestations*. These include carditis, arthritis, chorea, subcutaneous nodules, and erythema marginatum. The term "major" relates to the diagnostic importance and not to the frequency, or the severity, of the particular manifestation. Other signs and symptoms, while less characteristic, may still be helpful. These *minor manifestations* include fever, arthralgia, past history of rheumatic fever or rheumatic heart disease, prolongation of the P–R interval and positive acute phase reactants (ESR, CRP). Two major, or one major and two minor, manifestations indicate a high probability of rheumatic fever.

The Jones criteria were revised in 1965 to require evidence of a recent streptococcal infection to support the diagnosis of acute rheumatic fever[2]. There are two exceptions to this requirement: in some patients with Sydenham's chorea and in patients with insidious-onset carditis, streptococcal antibodies may have already returned to normal levels when the patient is first seen. The criteria were reviewed again in 1984 and no substantive changes were made (Table 6.1)[3].

The Jones criteria have proved useful in making comparable the series of different observers and in avoiding overdiagnosis. However, the pedantic and mindless application of the criteria may mislead. As Duckett Jones himself indicated, the criteria are only a guide, not a set of rules to be followed blindly. Also, one must admit that there are patients in whom the diagnosis

48

Table 6.1   Jones criteria (revised) for guidance in the diagnosis of rheumatic fever

Major manifestations	Minor manifestations
Carditis	Clinical
Polyarthritis	Fever
Chorea	Arthralgia
Erythema marginatum	Previous rheumatic fever or rheumatic heart disease
Subcutaneous nodules	
	Laboratory
	Acute phase reactions
	ESR, leukocytosis
	C-reactive protein
	Prolonged P–R interval

Plus supporting evidence of preceding streptococcal infection: increased ASO or other streptococcal antibodies; positive throat culture for group A streptococcus; recent scarlet fever.

From ref. 3

of rheumatic fever can neither be made nor excluded with certainty. In such cases it is better to make a diagnosis of *probable rheumatic fever* than arbitrarily to feign certainty.

Critique of the criteria

In the absence of a specific diagnostic test the criteria became widely accepted in many parts of the world. However, physicians in developing countries have found them less satisfactory than their Western colleagues[4]. The reasons for their criticisms were considered at a 1987 WHO Rheumatic Fever Study Group meeting, and their conclusions and recommendations are discussed below[5].

Arthralgia

A frequent criticism of the Jones criteria is that they are not sufficiently sensitive, and that children who have rheumatic fever may not be diagnosed and consequently go unprotected against recurrences. This criticism is heard most frequently in tropical countries where the clinical manifestations of rheumatic fever are said to differ from those in Western countries. Many physicians in developing countries believe that arthralgia merits recognition as a major manifestation because it is said to be more common than frank polyarthritis, in contrast to reports from Western countries[6,7]. This belief is based on retrospective reports from series of hospitalized patients with varying proportions of first attacks and recurrences.

Many factors can artificially decrease the incidence of joint involvement in hospitalized patients. Arthritis is an early, transient, and self-limited manifestation, and in areas where children are often seen late in the course of an attack the joint symptoms will have subsided. The distinction between polyarthralgia and polyarthritis can rarely be made with certainty from the history alone, since it is sometimes difficult to make this distinction even on physical examination. Also, the incidence of joint manifestations may be underestimated because patients with arthritis and no carditis are less likely to be admitted to hospitals when beds are at a premium.

That variations in the frequency of joint manifestations may be due to sampling biases is suggested by recent studies in several developing countries. In contrast to earlier reports, these were *prospective* studies limited to patients with an *initial* attack of rheumatic fever and, as noted in Table 6.2, the frequency[8-10] of polyarthritis was similar to that of Western countries[8-10]. In addition to such artificial variations there may be genuine ones, since the frequency of arthritis increases with age, and since the more severe the carditis, the greater the likelihood of mild or absent joint manifestations. Therefore, in countries where the afflicted children are younger and carditis is severe, joint manifestations may indeed be fewer, and transient arthralgia be more common than florid migratory polyarthritis.

The question of changing the Jones criteria to include arthralgia as a major manifestation was recently considered by the aforementioned WHO Rheumatic Fever Study Group[5]. It was felt that this change would increase the sensitivity of the criteria, but at the expense of specificity, and could lead to overdiagnosis. The latter would be less likely if the arthralgia was proved to have followed a streptococcal infection. Polyarthralgia plus a high ASO titer should always make one suspect rheumatic fever, and should be an indication for careful and repeated cardiac auscultation, as well as a search for other evidence of rheumatic fever.

Required evidence of a streptococcal infection

The main reason for the inclusion of a requirement for evidence of a prior streptococcal infection was to reduce the chances of overdiagnosis in patients with clinical syndromes which mimic rheumatic fever and fulfill the criteria, but are not preceded by a streptococcal infection[12].

At the time of the 1965 revision, WHO continued to recommend the earlier

Table 6.2   Frequency (percentages) of major manifestations in initial attacks of rheumatic fever recorded in prospective studies

	Kuwait[10]	*India*[8]	*Trinidad*[9]	*UK*[11]	*USA*[11]
Carditis	46	34	73	55	42
Polyarthritis	79	67	67	85	76
Chorea	8	20	3	13	8
Nodules	0.5	3	–	–	1
Erythema marginatum	0.5	2	–	–	4

version of the criteria, which did not insist on evidence of a preceding strepto-coccal infection. This was done because many countries lacked facilities to do streptococcal antibody tests. However, at present an ASO titer can be obtained in most centers throughout the world, and the WHO Rheumatic Fever Study Group recently recommended acceptance of the 1965 revised criteria. Unfortunately only 80% of acute rheumatic fever patients have an elevated ASO titer (the most commonly used antibody determination), but as more antibodies are determined, the more likely it is to find evidence of infection (see Figure 5.1). Anti-DNase B currently is the preferred "second test", but this test is still not available in many laboratories. Another test, streptozyme, has gained popularity as a "universal" streptococcal antibody test, but because of standardization problems the World Health Organiz-ation does not recommend the use of this test at the present time[13].

Insidious-onset carditis

It is fairly common in developing countries for patients to be seen for the first time with active carditis but with few or no other clinical or laboratory fin-dings of acute rheumatic fever. These patients often have a vague or no his-tory of prior rheumatic symptoms, but give a history of malaise, lethargy, poor appetite and the appearance of chronic illness for the past several months. They often first come to medical attention because of shortness of breath. On examination, signs of carditis are usually unmistakable. Such children have murmur(s), enlargement of the heart, and signs of congestive heart failure. Such patients may have only one major manifestation (carditis) or at most one major and one minor, such as low-grade fever or an elevated sedimentation rate. Therefore they do not fulfill the revised Jones criteria. Some experienced cardiologists have pointed out that as many as 25% of their rheumatic patients with active carditis have no history of rheumatic fever and insufficient other findings to meet the revised criteria[3]. Thus, strict adherence to the criteria would exclude such patients. This could be avoided if diagnosis of rheumatic fever were permitted in patients with late-onset, insidious-onset carditis, even in the absence of other rheumatic manifes-tations. Other forms of myocarditis must be excluded, and such patients must be distinguished from *inactive* valvular disease of presumed rheumatic origin. Ultrasound can be useful in confirming or excluding chronic valvular disease.

Diagnosis of recurrent attacks

Brief reference is made in Dr Jones' 1944 article to the diagnosis of rheumatic recurrences. He stated that "minor manifestations of rheumatic fever in the absence of other causation are presumptive evidence of rheumatic fever in patients with rheumatic heart disease."[1] This would suggest that he did not believe that the criteria need necessarily be fulfilled for the diagnosis of a rheumatic recurrence. However, neither the American Heart Association

1965 revision nor the 1984 review of the criteria make any reference to the diagnosis of recurrences of rheumatic fever[2,3]. A presumptive diagnosis of a recurrent attack should be allowed in patients with rheumatic heart disease or a reliable past history of rheumatic fever, who have only one major criterion *or* several minor criteria, *provided there is a significant change in the streptococcal antibody titer*. However, a firm diagnosis of a rheumatic recurrence should be made only after sufficient time has elapsed to exclude an intercurrent illness or a complication of rheumatic heart disease, such as infective endocarditis which can mimic a rheumatic recurrence.

The recommendations of the 1987 WHO Rheumatic Fever Study Group* can be summarized as follows: The latest revised Jones criteria should be adopted for general use but, in addition, the criteria should permit the diagnosis of rheumatic fever in the absence of two major or one major and two minor manifestations in patients with "pure" chorea, insidious or late-onset carditis, or rheumatic recurrence, after other possible causes have been excluded.

References

1. Jones, T. D. (1944). The diagnosis of rheumatic fever. *J. Am. Med. Assoc.*, **126**, 481
2. Jones criteria (revised) for guidance in the diagnosis of rheumatic fever. (1965). *Circulation*, **32**, 664
3. Jones criteria (revised) for guidance in the diagnosis of rheumatic fever. (1984). *Circulation*, **69**, 203A
4. Cherian, G. (1979). Acute rheumatic fever – the Jones criteria. A review and a case for polyarthralgia. *J. Assoc. Phys. India.*, **27**, 453
5. Rheumatic Fever and Rheumatic Heart Disease (1988). Report of a WHO Study Group. *WHO Technical Report Series*, Geneva: WHO (in press)
6. Padmavati, S. (1978). Rheumatic fever and rheumatic heart disease in developing countries. *Bull. WHO*, **56**, 543
7. Lue, H. C. *et al.* (1983). Clinical and epidemiologic features of rheumatic fever and rheumatic heart disease in Taiwan and the Far East. *Indian Heart J.*, **35**, 139
8. Sanyal, S. K. *et al.* (1974). The initial attack of acute rheumatic fever during childhood in North India: a prospective study of the clinical profile. *Circulation*, **49**, 7
9. Potter, E. V. *et al.* (1978). Tropical acute rheumatic fever and associated streptococcal infections compared with concurrent acute glomerulonephritis. *J. Pediatr.*, **92**, 325
10. Majeed, H. A. *et al.* (1981). Acute rheumatic fever during childhood in Kuwait. The mild nature of the initial attack. *Ann. Trop. Paediatr.*, **1**, 13
11. U.S.-U.K. Joint Report (1955). Rheumatic Fever Working Party. *Circulation*, **11**, 343
12. Laitinen, O. *et al.* (1975). Rheumatic fever and Yersinia arthritis. Criteria and diagnostic problems in a changing disease pattern. *Scand. J. Rheumatol.*, **4**, 145
13. World Health Organization (1986). Evaluation of the streptozyme test for streptococcal antibodies. *Bull. WHO*, **64**, 504

*The views of this international group of experts do not necessarily represent the decisions or the stated policy of the World Health Organization[5].

Chapter 7
Differential diagnosis

A number of conditions – some trivial, some serious – mimic rheumatic fever. They must be kept in mind and excluded before a definitive diagnosis of rheumatic fever is made. The conditions to consider vary, of course, with the clinical presentation.

The worst error is missing a serious disease which could have been cured effectively if diagnosed early (such as infective endocarditis, septic arthritis, or osteomyelitis).

Musculoskeletal conditions simulating rheumatic fever

Infectious arthritis
While infectious arthritis more commonly involves only one joint, it may be polyarticular and even migratory. Monoarticular involvement is uncommon in rheumatic fever, except in patients who have been treated with salicylates before other joints can flare. Virtually every infectious agent can localize in a joint and cause inflammation[1].

Among the pyogenic bacteria, the gonococcus is the most frequent cause of infectious arthritis in the Western world. Moreover, there is quite an overlap between the age preference of rheumatic fever and that of peak (and experimental) sexual activity – which predisposes to gonococcal infections. Therefore, the differential diagnosis between these two conditions comes up frequently, and is important.

We have found it useful to pay close attention to the localization of the disease at hand (in this we followed Osler: in his celebrated textbook he pointed out that vertebral, sternoclavicular, and phalangeal articulations are less often inflamed in acute rheumatic fever than in "gonorrhoeal rheumatism"). Tendons, tendineal sheaths, and sites of attachment of muscles to bone are much more frequently affected by gonococci than by rheumatic fever. Small purpuric spots or blisters should be looked for, especially on the extremities, as they are characteristic of disseminated gonococcal infection[2].

The history, of course, can help, but should not be overly relied upon (even now, after the sexual revolution of the 1960s, a young person may still be reluctant, afraid, or embarrassed to admit sexual activity). Gram stains and cultures are less likely to lie. If positive, they are very helpful.

Unfortunately, the synovial fluid is often negative for gonococci on Gram stain and on culture, even when the culture is done, as it should be, by plating the fluid on Thayer–Martin medium at the bedside of the patient or immediately after obtaining it. The gonococcus is very delicate, it dies off easily, and it's very fastidious; it needs a rich medium. A presumptive diagnosis is permissible even with a joint-tap negative for gonococci when gonococci are isolated from the portal of entry: the urethra, the rectum, or the pharynx. It is always prudent to exclude bacteremia by blood cultures.

Polyarthritis and polyarthralgia are frequent manifestations of infective endocarditis and in patients with pre-existing heart disease may be mistaken for a recurrence of rheumatic fever[3]. In the inner-city population of many American hospitals intravenous drug abusers are frequently seen with this syndrome, and early diagnosis is crucial to minimize the organ damage[4]. Osteomyelitis of the articular end of a bone can be difficult to distinguish from arthritis of the adjacent joint. Whenever an infectious agent is the suspected cause of arthritis, especially monoarticular arthritis, the joint involved should be tapped without delay for Gram stain and joint-fluid culture, and blood cultures should be obtained. Arthritis can occur also in conditions as diverse as meningococcemia, brucellosis, typhoid fever, tuberculosis, toxoplasmosis, and filariasis, to name a few.

Lyme disease
This interesting "new" disease, originally described in the Connecticut town that gave it its name, is being reported more and more from other locales and is probably world-wide – or, at least, common wherever trees are abundant and when ticks bite men. It has, at first blush, some similarities to rheumatic fever, in that it affects the skin, the heart, the joints, and the nervous system, but the similarity is more apparent than real and very seldom will cause confusion. The skin rash is *erythema chronicum migrans*, with few lesions which are much larger than those of *erythema marginatum* (although in later phases a rash similar to *erythema marginatum* may also be seen); early rheumatic complaints include migratory polyarthritis and tendinitis, but later the arthritis becomes localized to a few large joints and lasts longer than rheumatic fever. Chorea may appear; but other neurologic localizations are more frequent. The P–R interval may be prolonged but the characteristic murmurs of rheumatic fever are absent. A serologic test (antibody against the etiologic agent, *Borrelia burgdorferi*) is helpful[5].

Rheumatoid arthritis
When acute polyarthralgia or polyarthritis is the initial manifestation of this disease it can be easily confused with acute rheumatic fever. The age of onset sometimes provides a clue because polyarthritis in children under 3 years of age is almost never rheumatic fever, but may well be rheumatoid arthritis. The former condition should be suspected if many joints are involved at the

54

same time, and especially if there is symmetrical involvement – e.g. both knees or both wrists – or if there is finger joint, cervical spine, or temporomandibular joint involvement. Rheumatoid arthritis is also less migratory and less responsive to salicylates than is rheumatic fever. If joint pains persist for more than one week on an adequate amount of salicylates, then rheumatoid arthritis should be seriously considered. Morning stiffness is a helpful sign, but is less frequent in children than adults. Early in the course of acute rheumatoid disease, children will often develop an evanescent "salmon-pink" macular rash (which is not ringlike as that of erythema marginatum), splenomegaly, and lymphadenopathy, none of which occurs in acute rheumatic fever. Fever is often high and intermittent, with one or two swings a day in juvenile rheumatoid arthritis of systemic onset, while it is lower and remittent in rheumatic fever. Laboratory tests are not very helpful, but the chronic course of the arthritis in rheumatoid disease usually distinguishes it from rheumatic fever[6].

Reactive arthritis
Pain and swelling of the joints can be caused by a sterile synovial reaction to infections elsewhere in the body. A well-known example is severe hip pain associated with fever and upper respiratory infections in children, a benign clinical entity known as toxic synovitis of the hip. *Shigella* and *Salmonella* infections can also cause a reactive arthritis. In Scandinavian countries, *Yersinia enterocolitica* is currently a much more common cause of polyarthritis than rheumatic fever. *Yersinia* can apparently cause carditis also, adding to the diagnostic confusion[7].

Allergic conditions
The resemblance of serum sickness to rheumatic fever is well known. There can be confusion when patients with pharyngitis develop joint pains after treatment with penicillin, and the possibility of a penicillin reaction must be weighed against that of rheumatic fever occurring despite penicillin. The presence of hives, erythema multiforme, and angioneurotic edema strongly favors the diagnosis of a drug reaction. There can also be joint pains and swelling in the Henoch–Schönlein syndrome, but the appearance of purpuric lesions and their location over the lower half of the body usually settles the diagnosis.

Viral infections
Polyarthralgia and polyarthritis are known to occur in several types of viral infections. They occur in preicteric and anicteric viral hepatitis, and can be then recognized by the accompanying urticarial rash, abnormal liver function tests, low complement, and positive tests for hepatitis B surface antigen[8].

German measles (rubella) is another well-documented cause of arthritis, less common in children than in young adults. Joint symptoms can also occur following rubella vaccination[9]. The arboviruses are known causes of arthritis in some parts of the world, such as Africa and Australia (Chikungunyan and Onyongnyong arthritis). Other viral infections, such as mumps, rubella, and infectious mononucleosis, can also cause transient arthritis.

Hematologic disorders

Bone and joint pain due to malignant diseases can simulate rheumatic fever. As many as 10% of leukemic patients have such symptoms, at times even before the peripheral blood smear becomes abnormal. Leukemia should be suspected if there is an unusual degree of anemia or easy bruisability. A bone marrow examination is indicated in such patients.

Sickle-cell anemia and other hemoglobinopathies have many signs and symptoms in common with rheumatic fever: joint pains, heart murmurs, and abdominal pain. Loud apical systolic murmurs and cardiac enlargement may be secondary to chronic anemia and add to the diagnostic confusion. A sickle-cell preparation and hemoglobin electrophoresis will clarify the diagnosis. Other causes of chronic anemia, such as hookworm infestation, can also result in cardiac dilatation and functional heart murmurs from anemia that can be mistaken for organic heart disease.

Other miscellaneous "rheumatic" conditions

Children frequently complain of pain in the extremities. When there is not swelling or other signs of inflammation of the joints it may be difficult to determine whether the pain is in the muscle, bone, tendon, bursa, or within the joint. Muscle aches and pains commonly accompany or follow upper respiratory infections and are not to be confused with arthralgia. Pain behind the knees and in the muscles of the leg that awaken children at night (so-called growing pains) are not a manifestation of rheumatic fever, contrary to old belief. Limb pains are at times the expression of an emotional disorder.

Greenstick fractures and other traumatic injuries may masquerade as arthralgia. Orthopedic abnormalities of the feet may cause recurrent leg pains. Chondromalacia of the patella in adolescence is also a cause of pain, and at times even swelling around the knee. Osteochondroses of the hip (Legg–Calvé–Perthes disease) and of the upper end of the tibia (Osgood–Schlatter disease) can be confused with arthralgia.

Conditions simulating chorea

Abnormal movements due to other causes may be confused with Sydenham's chorea when there is no other evidence of rheumatic fever. Multiple tics or habit spasms are fairly easy to distinguish from choreiform movements. The former are repetitive and patterned and do not interfere with coordination. Hyperactive, fidgety children who cannot sit still and have short attention spans are sometimes erroneously said to have St Vitus' dance, the popular term for chorea.

Huntington's chorea rarely begins in childhood, and there is usually a strong family history. The movements associated with cerebral palsy are slower and more repetitive. Choreiform movements have been described in lupus erythematosus, following encephalitis from various causes and Wilson's disease and, as we have just mentioned, Lyme disease, but other features of these conditions are usually apparent.

Other common diagnostic errors

Fever
Protracted low-grade fever accompanied by vague aches and pains may lead to the suspicion of rheumatic fever. If in fact the fever is protracted, it is rarely due to rheumatic fever in the absence of other manifestations. Wide swings in fever are rare in rheumatic fever and are more suggestive of juvenile rheumatoid arthritis.

Abdominal pain
This complaint can precede other rheumatic manifestations and simulate an attack of appendicitis. However, rheumatic abdominal pain is diffuse. Vomiting is common in appendicitis and it does not usually occur early in the course of rheumatic fever. The pain and vomiting that occur after carditis and arthritis become apparent is due to liver congestion, or to salicylate or digitalis toxicity.

Streptococcal antibodies
Patients with illnesses that resemble rheumatic fever may by chance have an elevated ASO titer at the same time. An elevated titer is proof of a recent streptococcal infection but not of rheumatic fever, since most streptococcal infections are not followed by rheumatic fever.

Erythrocyte sedimentation rate
The erythrocyte sedimentation rate is elevated in a wide variety of inflammatory conditions and therefore is not diagnostic for rheumatic fever. It is a good screening test for inflammatory processes; in patients with joint symptoms or cardiac manifestations a normal sedimentation rate is evidence against acute rheumatic fever.

Cardiac conditions simulating rheumatic carditis and rheumatic heart disease

Innocent murmurs

Functional or innocent murmurs are frequently heard in children. They are always systolic in time, usually short, and are heard best over the pulmonic area or along the lower left sternal border. The pulmonic murmur is the most common. It is heard early in systole, is short, has an ejection quality (crescendo–decrescendo) and is separate from both first and second heart sounds. It is due to turbulence as blood passes through the pulmonary outflow tract. It is accentuated by high cardiac output states such as exercise, fever, anxiety, and anemia.

The parasternal innocent murmur, known also as Still's murmur, can occupy as much as two-thirds of systole. It is usually loudest in the third or fourth interspace just to the left of the sternum: usually grade 1 or 2, and occasionally even 3 on a scale of 6. In a thin child it is often audible at the apex, and even in the axilla. It is the quality, more than the loudness or transmission, that differentiates the parasternal innocent murmur from the organic murmur. The innocent murmur has a vibratory sound variously described as musical, groaning or twanging-string, and it lacks the characteristic blowing quality of the mitral regurgitation murmur.

Infective endocarditis

Infective endocarditis may be mistaken for a recurrent attack of rheumatic fever in patients with established rheumatic heart disease. Confusion is easy because infective endocarditis often affects the joints as well as the heart[3,4]. Joint involvement is more likely to be monoarticular, while rheumatic fever tends to affect more joints. High spiking fever is frequent in infective endocarditis, but not in rheumatic fever. The extracardiac manifestations of infective endocarditis, such as petechiae, splenomegaly, and hematuria, are useful in the differential diagnosis, but unfortunately tend to appear late in the course of the disease. Since missing or delaying the diagnosis of infective endocarditis can be disastrous, a high index of suspicion should be maintained and blood cultures should be done whenever there is a possibility of infective endocarditis.

Mitral valve prolapse

This is a common and usually benign disorder or anomaly (also called floppy mitral valve, click syndrome, or Barlow's syndrome) which can be confused with rheumatic mitral regurgitation and probably often was in the past. It can be distinguished from its rheumatic counterpart clinically on the basis of the characteristic systolic click and late systolic murmur. Echocardiography is the most reliable way to confirm the diagnosis. Mitral valve prolapse, like rheumatic heart disease, predisposes to infective endocarditis, though to a lesser extent[10].

Congenital heart disease

Acute rheumatic carditis is rarely mistaken for congenital heart disease, but chronic rheumatic valvular heart disease may be, and vice-versa. The systolic murmur of a ventricular septal defect due to a small left-to-right shunt can resemble the murmur of mild mitral regurgitation. Atrial septal defects associated with a deformed mitral valve can mimic rheumatic mitral regurgitation. There are a number of isolated defects of the mitral valve which are almost impossible to distinguish from rheumatic mitral regurgitation in the absence of a history of rheumatic fever. Prolapse of the mitral valve is a common cause of regurgitation. A mid-systolic click and late-systolic murmur are characteristic auscultatory findings. The sequelae of rheumatic fever may occasionally cause identical findings.

There are also non-rheumatic causes of the diastolic murmur of aortic regurgitation, which can occur in patients with ventricular septal defect and aortic insufficiency caused by congenital bicuspid aortic valve. Aortic valve disease without mitral valve involvement is rarely due to rheumatic fever, but not infrequently the aortic diastolic murmur persists, while the mitral one disappears.

Viral carditis

A number of viral agents, especially Coxsackie B and arboviruses, can cause myocarditis with cardiac enlargement, arrhythmias, and heart failure. The absence of a significant heart murmur generally excludes rheumatic fever as the etiology, although in recent years evidence of regurgitation obtained by Doppler ultrasound has been reported in the absence of significant murmur. However, a dilated heart from any cause can be associated with a murmur of mitral regurgitation. Viruses can also cause pericarditis. Viral pericarditis can be distinguished from rheumatic pericarditis since the latter does not occur without associated valvular involvement.

Viruses have been shown to cause valvulitis in experimental animals, and it was suggested that these agents can cause chronic valvular disease in humans. The proponents of this view believe that patients with acquired valvular disease and no history of rheumatic fever have been erroneously diagnosed as "silent" rheumatic carditis. It is certainly true that valvular heart disease can no longer be equated automatically with rheumatic heart disease when a history of arthritis and chorea is lacking. Valvular heart disease may be due to other etiologies, e.g., mitral valve prolapse. On the other hand, there is no conclusive proof that viruses can cause valvular disease in humans, and in countries where rheumatic fever is prevalent, and where the early manifestations of this disease are often overlooked because medical care is hard to obtain, patients with mitral insufficiency should be treated with anti-streptococcal prophylaxis even when a history of rheumatic fever is lacking. When there is also aortic regurgitation, there should be no doubt about a rheumatic etiology.

References

1. Goldenberg, D. L. and Reed, J. I. (1985). Bacterial arthritis. *N. Engl. J. Med.*, **312**, 764
2. Handsfield, H. H., Wiesner, P. J. and Holmes, K. K. (1976). Treatment of the gonococcal arthritis–dermatitis syndrome. *Ann. Intern. Med.*, **84**, 661
3. Doyle, E. F. *et al.* (1967). The risk of bacterial endocarditis during anti-rheumatic prophylaxis. *J. Am. Med. Assoc.*, **201**, 807
4. Churchill, M. A., Geraci, J. E. and Hunder, G. G. (1977). Musculo-skeletal manifestations of infective endocarditis. *Ann. Intern. Med.*, **87**, 754
5. Steere, A. C., Hutchinson, G. J., Rahn, D. W. *et al.* (1983). The spirochetal etiology of Lyme disease. *N. Engl. J. Med.*, **308**, 733
6. Taranta, A. (1988). JRA and red herrings. *Hosp. Pract.*, **23**, 129
7. Laitinen, O., Leiresalo, M. and Allander, E. (1975). Rheumatic fever and Yersinia arthritis. Criteria and diagnostic problems in a changing disease pattern. *Scand. J. Rheumatol.*, **4**, 145
8. Shumaker, J. B. *et al.* (1974). Arthritis and rash. *Arch. Intern. Med.*, **133**, 488
9. Cooper, L. Z. *et al.* (1969). Transient arthritis after rubella vaccination. *Am. J. Dis. Child.*, **118**, 218
10. Cheitlin, M. D. and Byrd, R. C. (1984). Prolapsed mitral valve: the commonest valve disease? *Curr. Probl. Cardiol.*, January

Chapter 8
Treatment

It is ironic that the field most important to a clinician – treatment – is the one that can boast the least progress. Indeed, there have been no significant advances in treatment since the first edition of this book was published. There is still no means to prevent damage to the heart when carditis occurs in the rheumatic patient. To be sure, surgery has provided relief for the most disabling end-results of carditis, but the outcomes are often imperfect, the operative mortality rate not negligible, and, whenever prostheses are used, the postoperative risk of infective endocarditis is significant, and perennial anti-coagulation is bothersome and not without risk. Nevertheless, surgical therapy of rheumatic heart disease has been a blessing to many, and should be considered in severe cases even when "rheumatic activity" seems to linger on[1,2]. There are now many more centers around the world doing cardiac surgery than there were seven years ago, but there is still a considerable backlog of patients in developing countries with advanced heart disease who remain on waiting lists for long periods of time. For surgical therapy, as for the medical therapy of established rheumatic heart disease, the reader is referred to textbooks of cardiology. We will deal here with the medical management of the acute attack.

General measures and bed rest

All patients with acute rheumatic fever should be placed at bed rest, if at all possible in a hospital, or otherwise at home. In either case, ideally they should be examined daily to detect valvulitis and to start treatment for heart failure promptly, should it appear. If carditis is going to occur, it will do so almost always within 2–3 weeks of onset, so that especially close observation is needed during this initial period. Thereafter, the duration and degree of bed rest vary with the nature and severity of the attack. Table 8.1 is a general guide. There are no controlled studies to support these recommendations, but they seem reasonable to us. The important point is that the regimen should be tailored to the disease manifestations of the particular patient, and a routine of prolonged restriction of physical activity should be avoided. In patients with carditis it may be difficult to tell when the rheumatic inflammatory process has become inactive. The acute phase reactants (ESR and CRP), are more helpful guides in the early stages of an attack than for judging the end of the active process. However, the CRP is the better of the two tests

61

Table 8.1   Guide for bed rest and ambulation in patients with acute rheumatic fever

Cardiac status	Management
No carditis	Bed rest for 2 weeks and gradual ambulation for 2 weeks even if on salicylates
Carditis, no cardiomegaly	Bed rest for 4 weeks and gradual ambulation for 4 weeks
Carditis, with cardiomegaly	Bed rest for 6 weeks and gradual ambulation for 6 weeks
Carditis, with heart failure	Strict bed rest for as long as heart failure is present and gradual ambulation for 3 months

From ref. 3

for this purpose, and if it is strongly positive it is likely that rheumatic activity is still present. A careful record of the pulse rate during sleep and at different levels of physical activity can provide a useful guide. A sleeping tachycardia should make one suspect that an active carditis is still present.

Antimicrobial treatment

Once the diagnosis of rheumatic fever has been established – but not before, lest other possible diagnoses be obscured – the patient should be started on penicillin, using either a single injection of 600,000 up to 1.2 million units of benzathine penicillin or 125–250 mg (200 to 400,000 units) of penicillin twice daily by mouth for 10 days. Patients who are allergic to penicillin should receive oral erythromycin, 20–40 mg/kg twice daily for 10 days. The purpose of this treatment is to eradicate streptococci that may still be in the pharynx before starting continual anti-streptococcal prophylaxis. Penicillin, however, or for that matter any other antimicrobial agent, does not have any effect on the clinical manifestations of acute rheumatic fever, the duration of the attack, or the prognosis. After the initial course of antibiotic therapy, long-term anti-streptococcal prophylaxis should be started.

Analgesic and anti-inflammatory treatment

Anti-inflammatory treatment is very effective in suppressing the acute inflammatory manifestations of rheumatic fever, so much so that prompt response of the arthritis to salicylates is helpful in supporting the diagnosis. More vigorous anti-inflammatory treatment, such as steroids, is useful in controlling pericarditis and the congestive failure of acute carditis; unfortunately, it has no effect on the long-term sequelae of active rheumatic fever; i.e., on the incidence of residual rheumatic heart disease[4,5]. A favorable response to steroids cannot be construed as confirming the diagnosis of rheumatic fever because most forms of arthritis, including septic arthritis, may "respond," at least initially, to steroids (although, of course, they should not be treated with them).

Anti-inflammatory drugs (salicylates and steroids) should be withheld if arthralgia or questionable arthritis is the only indication for suspecting rheumatic fever. This is particularly wise when the diagnosis is not definite, because pure analgesics, such as acetaminophen, will not interfere with the full development of migratory polyarthritis, the appearance of which may clinch the diagnosis, yet will control fever and make the patient comfortable.

Patients with definite clinical evidence of arthritis should be treated with aspirin: a total dose of 100 mg/kg/day, not to exceed 6 g per day, in divided doses for the first 2 weeks, and 75 mg/kg/day for the following 2–6 weeks. Sometimes slightly larger doses may be necessary to control arthritis. One should be alert to the possibility of salicylate intoxication, usually manifested by tinnitus (ringing in the ears) and hyperpnea.

In patients with carditis, especially if there is cardiomegaly or congestive failure, aspirin is often insufficient to control fever, discomfort, and tachycardia, or does so only at toxic or near-toxic doses. These patients should be treated with steroids. They improve clinically more rapidly than with salicylates[6]. Prednisone is the steroid of choice, starting with a dose of 2 mg/kg/day in divided doses not to exceed a total dose of 80 mg per day. In cases of extreme acuteness and severity, therapy should be started by intravenous administration of methylprednisolone (10–40 mg) followed by oral prednisone. After 2–3 weeks prednisone may be slowly withdrawn, decreasing the daily dose at the rate of 5 mg every 2–3 days. When tapering is started, aspirin at 75 mg/kg/day should be added and continued for 6 weeks after prednisone is stopped. This "overlap" therapy reduces the incidence of post-therapeutic clinical "rebounds" (i.e., reappearance of clinical manifestations shortly after treatment is stopped, or while it is being tapered, and without a new streptococcal infection which could have triggered a recurrence) (Table 8.2).

Steroids are recommended for patients with carditis because of the clinical impression that such patients tolerate steroids better and that congestive failure responds more rapidly than with salicylates. Most clinicians feel that death during the acute attack may be averted by steroid administration, but as far as long-term outcome is concerned, most well-controlled studies have

Table 8.2 Recommended anti-inflammatory agents for acute rheumatic fever

Clinical manifestation	Treatment
Arthralgia	Analgesics only
Arthritis	Salicylates 100 mg/kg/day for 2 weeks and 75 mg/kg/day for 4–6 weeks
Carditis	Prednisone 2 mg/kg/day for 2 weeks and taper of 2 weeks; salicylates 75 mg/kg/day at 2 weeks and continue for 6 weeks

failed to prove that the incidence of residual heart disease decreases after treatment with steroids, no matter what dosage is used or how long treatment is continued[4,5]. (In a disease as variable as rheumatic fever, conclusions cannot be drawn from uncontrolled observations.)

The termination of anti-inflammatory treatment may be followed in rheumatic fever patients by the reappearance within 2–3 weeks of laboratory abnormalities, or of clinical abnormalities as well. All the "laboratory rebounds" and most of the "clinical rebounds" are best left untreated, or should be treated symptomatically with analgesics or small doses of salicylates, lest the full treatment be followed by another rebound and the duration of the attack lengthened. Only the most severe clinical rebounds necessitate a second course of steroids.

In about 5–10% of all patients with rheumatic fever, ESR elevations persist for months after termination of therapy. This is a benign, unexplained phenomenon that should not alter the medical management. On the other hand, a persistently elevated C-reactive protein level often heralds a protracted course with subsequent flare-ups; these patients should be supervised closely. Once rheumatic fever has subsided and more than 2 months have gone by after stopping anti-inflammatory treatment, rheumatic fever will not reappear unless a new streptococcal infection occurs.

Diuretics and cardiotonic medication

The heart failure of rheumatic carditis is often controlled with bed rest and steroids only. If it is not, diuretics may be added first, followed by digitalis if needed. Digitalis should be used with caution because its therapeutic index may be decreased in rheumatic carditis. The need for digitalis should be re-evaluated at the end of the rheumatic attack, and periodically thereafter. In assessing the effect of digitalis, one should distinguish cardiac from emotional tachycardia, which subsides during sleep.

Treatment of chorea

Patients with chorea should be taken out of school and placed in a quiet environment at home, or preferably in a hospital. Bed rest is indicated for severe attacks and care must be taken to prevent the patient from bruising and falling out of bed. Since chorea often occurs as an isolated manifestation or a few months after arthritis or carditis, anti-inflammatory medication is not usually needed. Although steroids in large doses have been reported to control choreic movements it is difficult to be sure, because the course of chorea is unpredictable, and well-controlled studies are lacking. Since steroids (especially large doses) are not harmless, it would be unwise to use them in any but the most severe cases of chorea. Sedatives may be helpful early in the course of the illness and phenobarbital is the starting drug of choice (16–

32 mg every 6–8 h). If it is ineffective, haloperidol (0.01–0.03 mg/kg/day in two divided doses) or chlorpromazine (0.5 mg/kg every 4–6 h) may be tried. Patients with chorea, even in the absence of other manifestations, require long-term anti-streptococcal prophylaxis.

References

1. Kloth, H. H. *et al.* (1969). Open heart surgery and active rheumatic carditis. Report of a case. *Pediatrics*, **43**, 61
2. Barak, J. *et al.* (1984). Emergency mitral and aortic valve replacement during acute rheumatic fever in a 5-year-old child. *Scand. J. Thorac. Cardiovasc. Surg.*, **18**, 9
3. Markowitz, M. and Gordis, L. (1972). *Rheumatic Fever*, 2nd edn. Philadelphia: W. B. Saunders
4. U.K. and U.S. Joint Report on Rheumatic Heart Disease (1965). Ten-year report of a cooperative clinical trial of ACTH, cortisone and aspirin. *Circulation*, **32**, 457
5. Combined Rheumatic Fever Study Group (1965). A comparison of short-term intensive prednisone and acetylsalicylic acid therapy in the treatment of acute rheumatic fever. *N. Engl. J. Med.*, **272**, 63
6. Human, D. J. *et al.* (1984). Treatment choice in acute rheumatic carditis. *Arch. Dis. Child.*, **59**, 410

Chapter 9
Sequels of rheumatic fever: chronic rheumatic heart disease

Prognosis

The outcome of rheumatic fever spans the spectrum from complete recovery (always marred, however, by a predisposition to recurrences) to death from intractable heart failure during the acute attack. In between are the various kinds of chronic rheumatic heart disease, each with its own characteristic natural history, and with its own spectrum of severity.

Death during the first attack is unusual. In a large Western series of such cases the case fatality rate was about 1%[1]. In some series from developing countries the case fatality rates have been higher, but these series may have included recurrent attacks[2]. For recurrent attacks the mortality is much higher if the recurrences occur in patients with pre-existing heart disease and the heart is affected once again.

When a recurrent attack affects a patient previously free of heart disease the prognosis is very good, since heart disease rarely appears for the first time during a recurrent attack (Table 10.2, next chapter). By contrast, if a recurrent attack falls on an already damaged heart the effect can be devastating. Additional valve deformities may appear and refractory heart failure may develop. Polyarthritis, however painful, and chorea, however incapacitating, are always benign, and subcutaneous nodules and erythema marginatum, besides being benign even when florid, cause no discomfort at all. They are, in fact, signs more than symptoms, and must be looked for by the physician, lest they be missed.

The prognosis of rheumatic fever patients depends mainly on the manifestations present and on the severity of the initial attack. Patients with no carditis have the best prognosis, regardless of whether they have polyarthritis or chorea. Patients with chorea may develop mitral stenosis years after the attack of chorea[3].

Patients with carditis may eventually lose any clinically detectable evidence of heart disease (Table 9.1). Predictably, this favorable outcome is most common in patients with only questionable evidence of carditis during the acute attack – i.e., patients with mitral systolic murmur of doubtful organicity and doubtful or no cardiomegaly. It is still common in those with definite evidence of heart disease limited to one valve only – which is then

Table 9.1 Disappearance of murmur of mitral regurgitation after 5 or more years in patients maintained on continual monthly benzathine penicillin G

Reference country, year	Patient–years of follow-up	Recurrence rate per 100 patient-years	Disappearance of mitral murmur (%)
Tompkins (U.S.A., 1972)[4]	565	0.1	74
Thomas (England, 1961)[5]	365	1.3	58
Sanyal (India, 1982)[6]	425	0.6	65
Majeed (Kuwait, 1986)[7]	385	0.5	77

almost always the mitral valve – but less common still in those with multiple valvular involvement – usually the mitral and aortic valves. It is rare in those with marked cardiomegaly and congestive heart failure during the acute attack[8]. It is not uncommon to lose all evidence of involvement in one valve and to retain it in another – in particular, for the mitral valve to heal and the aortic valve to remain regurgitant[9].

Structural abnormalities of the valves and hypertrophy and dilatation of the heart may progress even in the absence of recurrences. Exactly how this comes about remains uncertain, but a vicious cycle of hemodynamic alterations is likely. Progressive scarring, including perhaps platelet aggregation, retraction, and calcification, plays a role[10].

Mitral regurgitation

As noted earlier, the diagnosis of mitral regurgitation is based on an apical systolic murmur with organic characteristics: loudness greater than grade two on a scale of six, duration throughout most of systole, blowing quality, transmission into the axilla, and persistence throughout changes of position and phases of respiration. When a patient with a murmur with some or all of these characteristics comes to medical attention without a history of rheumatic fever, other causes have to be considered as well. In recent years mitral valve prolapse has been recognized as a common cause of mitral regurgitation. It should be suspected if there is a mid-systolic click and the murmur is loudest late in systole. The diagnosis should be confirmed by echocardiography[11]. Congenital mitral regurgitation may also occur in the absence of mitral valve prolapse. The systolic murmur of a ventricular septal defect causing a small left to right shunt may also mimic rheumatic mitral regurgitation. In African countries where endomyocardial fibrosis is common, it can masquerade as rheumatic mitral regurgitation[12].

Mitral regurgitation always appears early in the acute attack. As noted earlier, it subsequently disappears in many patients maintained on diligent prophylaxis (Table 9.1). In other patients it may progress, even without recurrences ("mitral regurgitation begets mitral regurgitation") to advanced lesions. The progression is usually slow and patients tend to remain asymptomatic for many years and then begin to tire easily. At first the symptoms respond well to medical treatment, but later they may no longer respond; the mitral lesion can then be corrected surgically with good clinical results if left ventricular function has not deteriorated[13,14].

Echocardiography is valuable for assessing myocardial performance and defining hemodynamic abnormalities. As has already been noted, surgery can be carried out even if the rheumatic process is active, should the clinical state of the patient warrant it. A recent report described a successful mitral and aortic valve replacement in a 5-year-old child with acute rheumatic fever[15].

Aortic regurgitation

Aortic regurgitation also begins during the acute attack, but is usually detected somewhat later in the attack in patients who already have mitral regurgitation. The characteristic blowing "decrescendo" murmur along the left sternal border can easily be missed at first, when its duration is short. In patients who are found to have an aortic diastolic murmur and no history of rheumatic fever the additional presence of mitral regurgitation is a sure indication of rheumatic heart disease. When the aortic regurgitation is an isolated lesion, other causes have to be considered as well, such as syphilis, Marfan's syndrome, aortic valve anomalies, and infectious endocarditis. However, the combination of aortic and mitral regurgitation is a very strong indication of a rheumatic etiology.

A patient with rheumatic fever and aortic insufficiency may remain asymptomatic for years, but when symptoms occur they progress rapidly.

Mitral stenosis

Mitral stenosis does not appear *de novo* during the acute attack; it takes time to develop; many months and usually years. Detection of mitral stenosis during the acute attack, in fact, is considered evidence of a previous attack. Rheumatic fever is the only cause but one of mitral stenosis, the other being congenital mitral stenosis, which is rare, and manifests itself during infancy. The auscultatory findings consist of a rumbling apical diastolic murmur with presystolic accentuation and ending with a loud first sound. An accentuated second sound at the base, indicative of pulmonary hypertension, is often present. Atrial fibrillation is a frequent late complication; when it occurs there is no presystolic accentuation.

In the Western world mitral stenosis takes many years to develop and is mostly a disease of adult life. This is in striking contrast to the developing countries where mitral stenosis can develop rapidly and therefore often affects adolescents and even children as young as 5 years of age – "juvenile mitral stenosis"[16]. The interval between the appearance of rheumatic symptoms and tight mitral stenosis can be as short as 1 year[17].

Why mitral stenosis develops so fast in developing countries, and so slowly in the West, remains unclear. The occurrence of streptococcal infections and of acute rheumatic fever at a younger age may be a factor. Inadequate nutrition may impair the immune response and increase susceptibility to infections. (Other diseases also, notably measles, are more severe in developing countries – probably because of differences in nutrition.) Subclinical recurrent attacks of rheumatic fever may also play a role. In one Western series, mitral stenosis appeared only in patients with two or more recurrences, and in another large series of patients, who were maintained on regular monthly injections of benzathine penicillin for almost a decade, none developed mitral stenosis[4].

It is puzzling that even when rheumatic fever was common in the West, only a tiny minority of the patients undergoing commissurotomy were in their teens or younger, whereas in some developing countries as many as one-third of all commissurotomies are performed in patients under 20 years of age [18,19].

References

1. U.K. and U.S. Joint Report on Rheumatic Heart Disease (1965). The natural history of rheumatic fever and rheumatic heart disease. Ten-year report of a cooperative clinical trial. *Circulation*, **32**, 457
2. Lue, H. C. *et al.* (1983). Clinical and epidemiologic features of rheumatic fever and rheumatic heart disease in Taiwan and the Far East. *Indian Heart J.*, **35**, 139
3. Bland, E. F. (1961). Chorea as a manifestation of rheumatic fever: a long term perspective. *Trans. Am. Clin. Climatol. Assoc.*, **73**, 209
4. Tompkins, V. G. *et al.* (1972). Long term prognosis of rheumatic fever patients receiving regular intramuscular benzathine penicillin. *Circulation*, **45**, 543
5. Thomas, G. T. (1961). Five year follow-up on patients with rheumatic fever treated by bed rest, steroids or salicylates. *Br. Med. J.*, **1**, 1635
6. Sanyal, S. K. *et al.* (1982). Sequelae of the initial attack of acute rheumatic fever in children in North India. *Circulation*, **65**, 375
7. Majeed, H. A. *et al.* (1986). The natural history of acute rheumatic fever in Kuwait: A prospective six year follow-up report. *J. Chron. Dis.*, **39**, 361
8. Feinstein, A. R. *et al.* (1964). Rheumatic fever in children and adolescents. A long-term epidemiologic study of subsequent prophylaxis, streptococcal infections and clinical sequelae. VII. Cardiac changes and sequelae. *Ann. Intern. Med.*, **60** (Suppl. 5) 87
9. Spagnuolo, M. *et al.* (1971). Natural history of rheumatic aortic regurgitation. Criteria predictive of death, congestive heart failure, and angina in young patients. *Circulation*, **44**, 368
10. Selzer, A. and Cohn, K. E. (1972). Natural history of mitral stenosis: a review. *Circulation*, **45**, 878
11. DeMaria, A. N. *et al.* (1974). The variable spectrum of echocardiographic manifestations

of the mitral valve prolapse syndrome. *Circulation*, **50**, 33

12. Metras, D. M. *et al.* (1983). Endomyocardial fibrosis masquerading as rheumatic mitral incompetence. *J. Thorac. Cardiovasc. Surg.*, **86**, 753

13. Weinhouse, E. *et al.* (1982). Severe rheumatic mitral valve disease in children. Evaluation by echocardiography. *Pediatr. Cardiol.*, **3**, 197

14. John, S. *et al.* (1983). Mitral valve replacement in the young patient with rheumatic heart disease. Early and late results in 118 subjects. *J. Thorac. Cardiovasc. Surg.*, **86**, 209

15. Barak, J. *et al.* (1984). Emergency mitral and aortic valve replacement during acute rheumatic fever in a 5-year-old child. *Scand. J. Thorac. Cardiovasc. Surg.*, **18**, 9

16. Roy, S. B. *et al.* (1963). Juvenile mitral stenosis in India. *Lancet*, **2**, 1193

17. Paul, A. T. S. (1980). Closed mitral commissurotomy in children. In Borman, J. B. and Gotsman, M. S. (eds), *Rheumatic Valvular Disease in Children*. New York: Springer, pp. 126–148

18. Bailey, C. P. and Bolton, H. E. (1956). Criteria for and results of surgery for mitral stenosis. *N.Y. State J. Med.*, **56**, 825

19. Cherian, G. *et al.* (1964). Mitral valvotomy in young patients. *Br. Heart J.*, **26**, 157

Chapter 10
Rheumatic recurrences

Recurrences are one of the most common and important features of this disease, and make it different from most other diseases of infectious etiology. Before anti-streptococcal prophylaxis, 75% of rheumatic fever patients had one or more recurrent attacks during their lifetime, a major cause of the morbidity and mortality from this disease[1]. In countries where programs to prevent recurrences have been established, there has been a marked improvement in the natural history and prognosis of rheumatic fever. The methods available to prevent recurrences are discussed in Chapter 12.

Quantitative aspects

The tendency of rheumatic fever to recur is highest right after an attack and decreases thereafter, first sharply and then slowly. The decrease is due in part to the fact that most patients with first attacks of rheumatic fever are children, and that children are less and less prone to streptococcal infections as they grow older. It is also due to a decreasing tendency of streptococcal infections to elicit rheumatic fever as the child grows up (Figure 10.1) but especially as

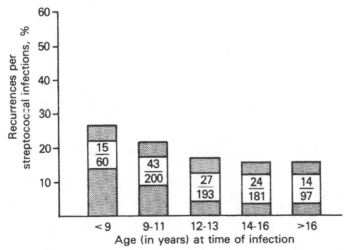

Figure 10.1 High recurrence rate per streptococcal infection in children, which decreases as the child grows up (from ref. 2)

71

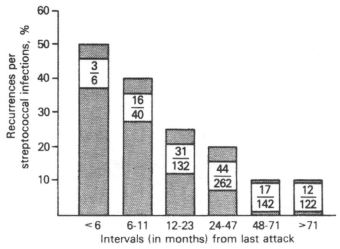

Figure 10.2 High recurrence rate per streptococcal infection in children, which decreases as the time interval since the latest rheumatic attack increases. Notice that this relationship is stronger than that with age of the child, shown in Figure 10.1 (from ref. 2)

the time interval since the first rheumatic attack becomes longer (Figure 10.2)[2]. Thus a child who has had a rheumatic fever attack within the last year has only an even chance (50% attack rate) of escaping rheumatic fever if his prophylaxis fails and a streptococcal infection breaks through. On the other hand, the patient who develops a streptococcal pharyngitis after 5 years of freedom from recurrences has nine chances out of ten (as the attack rate is only 10%). Hence the importance of prophylaxis for at least 5 years after an attack.

In addition to the time lapsed since the latest rheumatic fever attack, important risk factors associated with a high attack rate of rheumatic fever after a streptococcal infection are the presence of pre-established rheumatic heart disease (from a previous attack of rheumatic fever) and the vigor of the antibody response to streptococcal antigens. These two factors are independent of each other (Table 10.1)[3]. Moreover the clinical manifestations of the

Table 10.1 Ratio of rheumatic recurrences to streptococcal infections in patients stratified for pre-existing rheumatic heart disease and for ASO rise

ASO rise in number of tube dilutions	Pre-existing heart disease		No pre-existing heart disease	
0–1	3:24	(13%)	1:79	(1%)
2	10:38	(26%)	3:50	(6%)
3	6:16	(38%)	5:34	(15%)
4 +	9:16	(56%)	9:26	(35%)

From ref. 3

severity of streptococcal infection also correlate with the subsequent rheumatic fever attack rate per infection.

The precipitous decrease of the rheumatic fever recurrence rate per infection with time lapsed since the latest rheumatic fever attack makes one think that the initially high rate is the direct effect of the preceding attack. Conversely, the residual plateau of susceptibility (an attack rate close to 10% has been reported even after many years of freedom from rheumatic attacks) makes one think that it is the expression of an intrinsic susceptibility of the host, preceding even the first attack (and in fact determining it). As detailed elsewhere (section on etiology), there are additional reasons to believe that susceptibility to rheumatic fever indeed varies among humans according to genetically determined factors.

Qualitative aspects

The same clinical manifestations that were present in the initial attack of rheumatic fever tend to reappear in recurrent attacks. Conversely, manifestations that were absent in the first attack tend to be absent also in recurrent attacks. This is of particular importance in the case of carditis. Thus, a patient who has escaped carditis in the first attack is likely to remain free of rheumatic heart disease even if prophylaxis fails. The studies dealing with the outcome of recurrences in patients who did *not* have rheumatic heart disease during the first attack are summarized in Table 10.2[4]. In these patients the incidence of carditis during the recurrent attack, as well as the incidence of residual heart disease thereafter, is significantly lower than in those who had had carditis in the previous rheumatic attack[5,6]. The results of studies reported from developing countries are similar to the data from the United States. In a careful study of recurrences, by Majeed and his colleagues from Kuwait, the attack rate was highest during the first year following the initial episode[7]. These investigators also found that, if the patient escapes carditis in the initial attack, he will likely continue to do so in subsequent recurrences. Similar results were obtained by Sanyal in Indian patients[8].

Table 10.2 Incidence of carditis in patients with recurrent rheumatic fever who had *not* acquired heart disease in their previous attack

Reference	No. of patients with recurrence	No. of patients with RHD thereafter
Boone and Levine, 1938	68	4 (6%)
Feinstein and Spagnuolo, 1960	71	10 (14%)
Kuttner and Mayer, 1963	50	6 (12%)
U.K.–U.S. Cooperative Study, 1964	10	0
Sanyal *et al.*, 1982	14	1 (7%)
Majeed *et al.*, 1983	26	2 (8%)

From refs 4, 5, 7, and 8

References

1. Roth, I. R. *et al.* (1937). Heart disease in children. A rheumatic group. I. Certain aspects of age of onset and of recurrences in 488 cases of juvenile rheumatism. *Am. Heart. J.*, **13**, 36
2. Spagnuolo, M. *et al.* (1971). The risk of rheumatic recurrences after streptococcal infections. Prospective study of clinical and social factors. *N. Engl. J. Med.*, **285**, 641
3. Taranta, A. *et al.* (1964). Relation of rheumatic fever recurrence rate per streptococcal infection to the titers of streptococcal antibodies. *Ann. Intern. Med.*, **60** (Suppl. 5) 47
4. Taranta, A. and Markowitz, M. (1981). *Rheumatic Fever: A guide to its recognition, prevention and cure with special reference to developing countries.* Lancaster, England: MTP Press
5. U.K.–U.S. Joint Report (1960). The evolution of rheumatic heart disease in children. *Circulation*, **22**, 503
6. Tompkins, D. G. *et al.* (1972). Long term prognosis of rheumatic fever patients receiving regular intramuscular benzathine penicillin. *Circulation*, **45**, 543
7. Majeed, H. A. *et al.* (1986). The natural history of acute rheumatic fever in Kuwait: a prospective six-year follow-up report. *J. Chronic Dis.*, **39**, 361
8. Sanyal, S. K. *et al.* (1982). Sequelae of the initial attack of rheumatic fever in children in North India. A prospective five-year follow-up study. *Circulation*, **65**, 375

Chapter 11
Prevention of recurrent attacks

Prophylaxis of recurrences is the finest achievement of medicine in rheumatic fever. It is markedly effective and, in fact, it practically eliminates recurrences if injectable benzathine penicillin G is used. However, a great deal of patience, perseverance, and persuasiveness are required on the part of the health personnel involved. The success of secondary prophylaxis is way out of proportion to the numerical reduction of rheumatic fever attacks, because recurrences cause a disproportionate number of deaths and disabilities. Actually, the change in morbidity and mortality of the disease in the Western world is largely due to the reduction of recurrences.

Many developing countries have established secondary prevention programs. In a cooperative study carried out by the World Health Organization, a significant decline in hospitalization rates among patients on prophylaxis was demonstrated[1]. In Taiwan the 8-year mortality rate among rheumatic patients on prophylaxis was 3% compared to 28% among patients without prevention (Table 11.1)[2].

Continual parenteral prophylaxis

Intramuscular long-acting benzathine penicillin G (BPG) is by far the most effective prophylactic drug (Figure 11.1)[3]. It is the treatment of choice for all patients who are not allergic to penicillin, and especially for high-risk patients – that is, those with heart disease, multiple previous attacks, or those unlikely to take daily oral medication.

The recommended dose of BPG is 1.2 million units by intramuscular injection every 4 weeks. The original, as well as confirmatory, prevention

Table 11.1 Changes in mortality rates after long-term chemoprophylaxis

Study period	Without prevention			On prevention		
	No. of patients	Average years follow-up	Died (%)	No. of patients	Average years follow-up	Died (%)
1946–60	49	5	24.5	–	–	–
1961–75	101	8.4	28.7	131	5.5	3.1
1976–81	–	–	–	124	3.5	2.4

From ref. 2

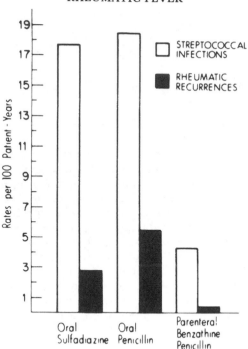

Figure 11.1 Streptococcal infection rates and rheumatic fever recurrence rates per 100 patient-years for three prophylactic drug regimens (from Taranta, A. and Gordis, L. (1972). The prevention of rheumatic fever. *Cardiovasc. Clin.*, **4**, 1)

studies in the United States found this regimen virtually eliminated recurrences in children and adolescents who received their injections on schedule (Table 11.2). Data from countries such as India and Taiwan indicate a slightly lower, but still very good, level of effectiveness[4,5]. However, recently, physicians in some developing countries have been recommending an injection every 3 weeks[6]. One controlled study of a small group of patients showed a significant difference in the recurrence rates when the two regimens were compared[7]. Since some patients do not have detectable serum levels of penicillin during the final week following a single intramuscular dose, it is possible that a 3-week schedule may be more effective when there is unusually heavy exposure to streptococci and/or the individual is at greater risk of infection for other reasons[8]. Therefore, it may be desirable to administer BPG every 3 weeks in *selected* patients. The potential advantage of a more frequent schedule must be weighed against the potential risk of higher drop-out rates because of the added inconvenience and cost.

Care must be taken in selecting the best site for injection, which most authorities agree is the buttocks, except in children under 2 years of age, for whom the upper or mid-lateral thigh is preferable. As with any intramuscular

Table 11.2   Rheumatic fever recurrence rate in patients receiving benzathine penicillin G every 4 weeks

Reference year, country	No. of patients	Patient-years follow-up	Recurrence per 100 patient-years
Stollerman (1955), U.S.A.[9]	145	241	0
Wood (1964), U.S.A.[3]	146	560	0.4
Tompkins (1972), U.S.A.[10]	115	1,073	0.1
Lue et al. (1982), Taiwan[2]	182	513	1.7
Sanyal et al. (1982), India[4]	65	425	0.6
Neutze (1984), New Zealand[11]	228	399	1.5

injection, meticulous attention also must be paid to avoiding an intra-arterial injection by pulling back on the plunger to make certain that the needle is not in a blood vessel[12]. There can be persistent pain for 1 or 2 days at the site of injection of BPG. Recent improvements in the preparation have made this less of a problem. The incidence and severity of pain can be significantly reduced by the addition of procaine penicillin G to the BPG preparation[13]. However, if this is done the total dose of BPG should not be reduced. It has been our experience that the discomfort becomes more tolerable with repeated injections of BPG, and rarely does the drug have to be discontinued for this reason. (The nature and incidence of allergic reactions are discussed later in this chapter.)

Continual oral prophylaxis

Sulfadiazine is the drug of choice for the exceptional patient who will not tolerate injections, or who is truly allergic to penicillin. The dose is 0.5 g once daily in children weighing less than 30 kg, and 1.0 g for older children and adults. Although reactions are rare, a blood count is advised after the first few weeks and the drug should be discontinued if the white blood cell count falls below 4000 and the neutrophil level below 35%. The patient should be advised to watch for skin rashes.

Oral penicillin can be used, but is somewhat less effective than sulfadiazine. The dose is 125 mg (200,000 units) twice a day. In contrast to sulfadiazine, a month's supply of oral penicillin costs more than a single dose of BPG. Another disadvantage is that oral penicillin causes the emergence of resistant alpha-streptococci in the mouth, whereas BPG and sulfadiazine do not[14]. Resistant alpha-streptococci in the oral cavity are a potential hazard for patients with rheumatic heart disease because these bacteria may cause infective endocarditis[15].

The major drawback of any oral medication for continual prophylaxis is the problem of compliance, which may be poor even when the patient seems to be cooperative. BPG by injection overcomes this problem as long as the patient comes to the clinic or the doctor's office.

Duration of continual prophylaxis

The risk of a recurrence is greatest during the first 3–5 years after an attack. Therefore every effort should be made to maintain prophylaxis during this critical period as a minimum in *all* patients. However, prophylaxis should be continued whenever possible beyond this period, at least into adult life, past the early childbearing years when children are certain to bring streptococci into the home. Reduction of the duration of prophylaxis to 5 years has been suggested for patients who have escaped carditis during the initial attack, since carditis is unlikely, should there be a recurrence[16]. However, there is general agreement that, if there is residual heart disease, prophylaxis is recommended for the lifetime of the patient.

As mentioned earlier, in some patients the diagnosis of rheumatic fever must be probable rather than definite rheumatic fever. In such cases the length of prophylaxis can be shortened in proportion to the doubts the physician has on the diagnosis.

Obstacles to continual prophylaxis

In theory the prevention of recurrent attacks should be a simple matter. The population at risk is a well-defined group, and highly effective drugs are available. In practice, however, there are many obstacles which stand in the way, especially in countries with limited resources. The following sections comment on some of the obstacles and suggest recommendations to overcome them.

Delay in diagnosis

It is a common experience in many developing countries to see children who already have advanced heart disease at the time of their first medical contact[17]. Prophylaxis of recurrence can do little to alter the poor prognosis in

Table 11.3 Antimicrobial therapy to prevent recurrences of rheumatic fever

Medication	Dosage
Benzathine penicillin G	1.2 million units IM every 3–4 weeks
Sulfadiazine (oral)	⩽ 30 kg weight: 0.5 g/day
	> 30 kg weight; 1.0 g/day
Penicillin (oral)	125 mg (200,000 units) twice daily

many of these patients.

Delay in diagnosis is due mainly to lack of easy accessibility to medical care. Also, in the absence of arthritis or chorea, the parents may not recognize that the child is sick until frank heart failure appears. Still another reason is that primary-care physicians are not sufficiently alert to the early signs of rheumatic fever. Children with arthralgia, or with a suspicious murmur, should be followed up closely.

Failures in follow-up

Rheumatic fever is mainly a disease of the poor, most of whom are not under regular medical care. For this population, follow-up is a major problem; drop-out rates are often exceedingly high. Therefore, to be effective, a rheumatic fever prevention program must have a system for following up patients who do not return for their appointments, and for restoring them to regular care. Hospital rheumatic clinics do not usually have the personnel to go into the community to locate and recall such patients. Once a non-compliant patient is identified, the public health or school health nurse, the home health visitor, community health aide or village worker, if such are available, should be notified. Not only are these individuals already out in the community, but they often relate better to families than hospital personnel and are more likely to restore reluctant patients to regular prophylaxis. (See Chapter 13, "Role of health care workers other than physicians in the control of rheumatic fever.")

In the clinic of one of the authors a diligent patient was used to track down and bring back to the clinic those patients who skipped appointments (the diligent patient was called a "skip-tracer"); also a club was organized ("the mending hearts club") to favor a positive identification with the clinic and to allay anxieties and dispel confusion by group discussions.

Cost of medication

The cost of medication is still another reason for discontinuing medication. A pilot project in the Philippines showed a significant decrease in drop-out and recurrence rates among patients who received BPG free of charge compared with patients who had to pay[18]. Hospitals and community health centers with organized rheumatic fever follow-up programs should have an uninterrupted supply of medication and, if needed, a government subsidy to cover the cost. The additional burden for national treasuries would be small compared with the expanding numbers and growing costs of cardiac operations performed in government hospitals on patients with advanced rheumatic heart disease.

Fear of penicillin reactions

There are still many physicians in developing countries who are fearful of allergic reactions to penicillin, and this has deterred them from maintaining patients on long-term prophylaxis. However, allergic reactions to BPG are neither more frequent nor more severe than following treatment with any other penicillin compound given parenterally at the same dose. Furthermore, when allergic reactions do occur following the use of BPG, they are usually transient, even though penicillin remains in the tissues and in the bloodstream. It has been postulated that this is due to the formation of protective blocking antibodies that compete for the penicillin-derived antigens and prevent them from combining with sensitizing antibodies[19].

Studies of antibodies to penicillin in children on long-term benzathine penicillin G reveal that a large percentage develop IgG antibodies to penicillin and a much smaller number develop IgE antibodies. The latter are believed to be responsible for immediate reactions, including anaphylactic shock. However, none of the children with IgG or IgE antibodies developed clinical signs of penicillin allergy[20].

Allergic reactions in children have been infrequent and mild, mainly urticaria and occasionally serum sickness. In the original study using BPG to prevent recurrences of rheumatic fever, there were five mild reactions among 410 children who had received 4871 injections over a period of several years[9]. Subsequent studies have shown equally mild reactions and very low rates of reaction.

Allergic reactions are more frequent, and are likely to be more severe, in adults than in children. In one study among military personnel, 23 out of 2100 adults, but only 1 of 2200 of their children, suffered reactions[21]. In another study of 76,000 adults, 0.85% had reactions and 0.65% were severe[22]. There were no deaths in this large group, but fatal reactions have been reported in adults. In a U.S. national survey of 94,655 adults treated in venereal disease clinics, moderate-to-severe reactions occurred in 0.025% and one patient died[23]. Fatalities have been reported following the use of BPG in four adult rheumatic patients[24,25]. Each of these patients was being treated for congestive heart failure, and non-allergic causes of death could not be excluded entirely.

Although the authors know of no documented fatalities among *children* receiving BPG for rheumatic prophylaxis, we have encountered anecdotal reports of such occurrences from practicing physicians in developing countries. The actual number of such fatalities, the type of penicillin used, and the clinical circumstances at the time of the injection need to be documented. It is noteworthy that among the many reports of secondary prevention programs in developing countries, no mention is made of serious allergic reactions.

What precautions should be taken to prevent allergic reactions? If there is a clear-cut history of a previous allergic reaction to penicillin, then alternative therapy, such as sulfadiazine, should be used instead. It is an entirely satisfactory prophylactic agent if taken every day. The time and expense of routine skin-test screening for penicillin allergy does not appear warranted for children. In the United States, routine skin testing is not done in history-negative patients, even when they are adult. However, if there is an extraordinary fear of penicillin reactions because of alleged fatalities in a community, and skin testing has been the customary method for screening patients, then physicians may feel compelled to do skin testing. Unfortunately, skin testing with dilute aqueous penicillin, which is the method most often used, will not identify all patients with potentially serious reactions. In fact, minimal reactions to such skin testing are often over-interpreted, and this needlessly denies using optimal antibiotic therapy. A derivative of penicillin, penicylloyl-polylsine, which is available commercially, used in conjunction with aqueous penicillin G, increases the chances of identifying allergic patients[26]. Another penicillin derivative, so-called minor determinents mixture, increases the predictive value of skin testing to detect individuals at risk of developing anaphylaxis, but unfortunately this material is not available commercially[27].

Whichever agent is used, a scratch test should be done first with one drop of the reagent on the abraded skin. Tests are read after 15 min and a positive reaction is defined as a wheal with a surrounding zone of erythema 3 mm or greater in diameter. Negative responders should be tested intradermally with 0.5 ml of reagent. After 15 min a positive reaction is read as a wheal of erythema 1–2 mm greater than the initial bleb.

To sum up, while an allergic reaction to penicillin can never be entirely avoided, serious reactions are rare, especially in individuals under 20 years of age. In countries where rheumatic fever causes as many as 25–40% of all cases of heart disease, the benefits of prevention with benzathine penicillin far outweigh the risk of serious reactions.

Mass prophylaxis

Mass prophylaxis with antimicrobial agents was first used in U.S. military camps during and following World War II to effectively bring epidemics of streptococcal pharyngitis and rheumatic fever under control. Military bases were plagued by such outbreaks, and this led to the routine of administering one injection of benzathine penicillin G to every recruit upon arriving at the camp[28,29]. Rheumatic fever virtually disappeared thereafter. This routine was discontinued about 1980 because of the general decline in rheumatic fever nationally. However, the recent resurgence of rheumatic fever in the United States, noted in earlier chapters, included an outbreak in a naval base where within a short period of time the rheumatic fever attack rate jumped from 0.75 to 80/100,000 recruits[30]. Mass prophylaxis with an injection of benzathine penicillin G for every incoming recruit has been reinstituted.

The use of mass prophylaxis in civilian populations has been limited to outbreaks confined to schools and to other institutions with defined population groups[31].

References

1. Strasser, T. *et al.* (1981). Report of a WHO international cooperative project. *Bull. WHO*, **59**, 285
2. Lue, H. C. *et al.* (1983). Clinical and epidemiological features of rheumatic fever and rheumatic heart disease in Taiwan and the Far East. *Indian Heart J.*, **35**, 139
3. Wood, H. F. *et al.* (1964). Rheumatic fever in children and adolescents. III. Comparative effectiveness of three prophylactic regimens in preventing streptococcal infections and rheumatic recurrences. *Ann. Intern. Med.*, **60**, (Suppl. 5), 31
4. Sanyal, S. K. *et al.* (1982). Sequelae of the initial attack of acute rheumatic fever in children from North India. *Circulation*, **65**, 375
5. Lue, H. C. *et al.* (1979). The natural history of rheumatic fever and rheumatic heart disease in the Orient. *Jpn Heart J.*, **20**, 237
6. Saran, R. K. *et al.* (1985). Is monthly injection of benzathine penicillin adequate for rheumatic fever prevention in our country? *J. Assoc. Physicians India*, **33**, 641
7. Lue, H. C. *et al.* (1986). Rheumatic fever recurrences: Controlled study of 3-week versus 4-week benzathine penicillin prevention programs. *J. Pediatr.*, **108**, 299
8. Lade, R. I. *et al.* (1958). Concentration of penicillin in the serum following intramuscular administration of benzathine penicillin G to children with inactive rheumatic fever. *Pediatrics*, **67**, 387
9. Stollerman, G. H. *et al.* (1955). Prophylaxis against group A streptococci in rheumatic fever. The use of a single monthly injection of benzathine penicillin. *N. Engl. J. Med.*, **259**, 581
10. Tompkins, D. G. *et al.* (1972). Long term prognosis of rheumatic fever patients receiving regular intramuscular benzathine penicillin. *Circulation*, **45**, 543
11. Neutze, J. M. (1984). Rheumatic fever: an unsolved problem in New Zealand. *NZ Med. J.*, **97**, 592
12. Stoller, K. P. and Losey, R. (1985). Inadvertent intra-arterial injection of penicillin: an unseen danger. *Pediatrics*, **75**, 785
13. Krugman, S. and Powell, V. E. (1956). Local tolerance to penicillin: a comparison of five intramuscular preparations. *J. Pediatr.*, **49**, 699
14. Sprunt, K. *et al.* (1968). Penicillin resistant alpha streptococci in the pharynx of patients given oral penicillin. *Pediatrics*, **42**, 957
15. Doyle, E. F. *et al.* (1967). The risk of bacterial endocarditis during anti-rheumatic prophylaxis. *J. Am. Med. Assoc.*, **201**, 807
16. Majeed, H. A. *et al.* (1984). Recurrences of acute rheumatic fever: a prospective study of 79 episodes. *Am. J. Dis. Child.*, **138**, 341
17. Fadahuni, H. O. (1981). Rheumatic fever in Nigerian children: a prospective study. *Ann. Trop. Paediatr.*, **1**, 115
18. Bravo, L. C. *et al.* (1979). Streptococcal infections and rheumatic recurrences in subjects on secondary prophylaxis. *Philippine J. Int. Med.*, **17**, 12
19. Peter, G. and Dudley, M. N. (1985). Clinical pharmacology of benzathine penicillin G. *Pediatr. Infect. Dis.*, **4**, 586
20. Strannegard, I. L. *et al.* (1987). Antibodies to penicillin in children receiving long-term secondary prophylaxis for rheumatic fever. *Allergy*, **42**, 502
21. Schneider, W. F. *et al.* (1964). Prevention of streptococcal pharyngitis among military personnel and their dependents by mass prophylaxis. *N. Engl. J. Med.*, **270**, 1205
22. Frank, P. F. *et al.* (1965). Protection of a military population from rheumatic fever. *J. Am. Med. Assoc.*, **193**, 775
23. Rudolph, A. H. and Price, E. V. (1973). Penicillin reactions among patients in venereal disease clinics. *J. Am. Med. Assoc.*, **223**, 499
24. Hsu, I. and Evans, J. M. (1958). Untoward reactions to benzathine penicillin G in a study of rheumatic fever prophylaxis in adults. *N. Engl. J. Med.*, **259**, 581
25. Steigmann, F. and Suker, J. R. (1962). Fatal reactions to benzathine penicillin G: Report of three cases and discussions of contributing factors. *J. Am. Med. Assoc.*, **179**, 288

26. Solley, G. O. *et al.* (1982). Penicillin allergy: clinical experience with a battery of skin tests. *J. Allergy Clin. Immunol.*, **69**, 238
27. Erffmeyer, J. E. (1986). Penicillin allergy. *Clin. Rev. Allergy*, **4**, 171
28. Morris, A. J. and Rammelkamp, C. H. (1957). Benzathine penicillin G in the prevention of streptococcal infections. *J. Am. Med. Assoc.*, **165**, 664
29. Davis, J. and Schmidt, W. C. (1957). Benzathine penicillin G: Its effectiveness in the prevention of streptococcal infections in a heavily exposed population. *N. Engl. J. Med.*, **256**, 339
30. *Morbidity and Mortality Weekly Report* (1988). Acute rheumatic fever at a Navy Training Center, **37**, 7
31. Zimmerman, R. A. *et al.* (1962). An epidemiologic investigation of a streptococcal and rheumatic fever epidemic in Dickensen, North Dakota. *Pediatrics*, **30**, 712

Chapter 12
Prevention of first attacks of rheumatic fever

The prevention of recurrences is very useful indeed to patients after a first attack of rheumatic fever but will never, by definition, eradicate the disease from the population at large. Moreover, many children suffer severe, irreversible heart damage from their first attack of rheumatic fever: to them the triumphs of secondary prophylaxis are no consolation. In some countries it is acknowledged that "the initial attack of acute rheumatic fever is hardly ever diagnosed in our environment. In most cases... cardiac damage is already severe and death from cardiac failure, common"[1]. Hence the importance of preventing first attacks (primary prevention). Well-controlled studies in military populations have shown that 90% of first attacks can be prevented by adequate antibiotic treatment of the preceding streptococcal pharyngitis[2] (see Table 2.1, p.10).

Prevention of first attacks of rheumatic fever involves the detection and treatment of streptococcal pharyngitis and, unlike secondary prevention, must be directed at the general population, especially for individuals between 3 and 20 years of age, the age span at highest risk for rheumatic fever. It requires general education about the importance of treating sore throats in children, and adequate resources to deliver good primary care for the general population. Some developing countries are establishing primary care networks to reach the general population. Costa Rica, in Central America, is a good example of what can be accomplished[3]. A national system of primary care was established in 1970, coupled with professional and educational programs directed at treating all respiratory infections in children to prevent rheumatic fever, i.e., each child with an upper respiratory infection coming to a health center was given an injection of BPG. By 1980 the number of rheumatic fever admissions to the Children's Hospital had been drastically reduced from over 100 annually to fewer than 10.

Diagnosis of streptococcal pharyngitis

The "classic" picture of a "strep" sore throat includes the fairly rapid onset of moderate-to-high fever followed by pain on swallowing; a fiery red pharynx with yellowish patches of exudate; and tender, enlarged anterior cervical lymph glands. There is also often headache and abdominal pain. Tender, enlarged glands and exudate are the most suggestive signs of a streptococcal infection. A fine, red, granular eruption of scarlet fever is diagnostic for a streptococcal infection.

Pharyngitis due to a viral infection has a more insidious onset and the throat feels "scratchy" or irritated. Viral upper respiratory infections are generally not limited to pharyngeal findings and include other signs and symptoms such as coryza, cough, and hoarseness. Vomiting and diarrhea may also occur. The presence of vesicles and/or ulcers in the pharynx strongly suggests a viral etiology. Viral infections may be accompanied by a macular eruption which is to be differentiated from the rash of scarlet fever.

Table 12.1 summarizes the diagnostic clues pointing to a viral or streptococcal etiology[4].

The distinction between streptococcal and viral pharyngitis is virtually impossible if redness of the pharyngeal tissues is the only finding on physical examination. Very often this is the case, especially in tropical climates where the classical syndrome of streptococcal pharyngitis is reported to be uncommon[5,6]. When the diagnosis is in doubt, which is in most of the cases, the throat should be cultured if appropriate facilities are available and affordable. Throat cultures are of considerable help, and have been used extensively in affluent countries for the past 30 years. The cost of a throat culture can be kept down if the request from the laboratory is limited to identifying the presence or absence of beta-hemolytic streptococci, and if the many bacteria which make up the normal flora are disregarded.

Methods are now available for rapid (i.e., 10 min) bacteriologic confirmation by antigen detection tests directly from the throat swab[7]. The drawbacks of these tests are that they are more expensive and less sensitive than the traditional throat culture. They are not recommended for general use at this time, but as the technology improves, antigen detection tests may replace

Table 12.1 Comparison of features of streptococcal and viral pharyngitis

	Streptococcal	Viral
Season	Winter and Spring (U.S.A.) rainy months (tropics)	Varies with agent
Age	3–20 years	All ages
Onset	Often abrupt	More gradual
Initial symptoms	Pain on swallowing	"Scratchy" sore throat
Pharyngeal appearance	Redness, edema, patchy, yellow exudate	Redness, ulcers, vesicles ± exudate
Cervical nodes	Enlarged, tender	May or may not be enlarged
Other symptoms	Headache, abdominal pain	Coryza, cough, hoarseness, diarrhea
Skin	Fine, red rash (scarlet fever)	Macules, papules, vesicles

the throat culture. It should also be noted that streptococcal antibody determinations are of no diagnostic value during the acute stage of a streptococcal infection, since it takes at least 1–2 weeks after the infection to detect a rise in antibodies.

Technique of taking a throat culture

The throat culture should be taken before antibiotic therapy. The tongue should be depressed, the throat should be clearly visualized and well lit, the swab must be rubbed vigorously over each tonsillar area without touching the tongue or the lips. The swab is then sent to a laboratory, according to the laboratory's instructions, or it may be streaked directly on a blood agar plate. The plate is read after overnight incubation.

Diagnosis without a throat culture

In many locations where patients with sore throats need medical attention, throat cultures are just not available or not affordable. In other locations, such as the busy emergency room of a large city hospital, it may be unwise to wait for the result of the throat culture even if it were available, since the physician may suspect that the patient will not come back to be treated (or not treated) the day after, on the basis of the culture result. One then may have to treat "either now or never." In such cases (and they are the majority in the world at large) the diagnosis will have to be made on the general basis of the clinical clues outlined above (Table 12.1). It should be noted that, in addition to the findings of the patient at hand, the diagnosis should be influenced by the prevalence of streptococcal infections and of its sequelae in the community: the more prevalent these diseases, the more likely the diagnosis in an individual patient.

If the patient is treated on clinical suspicion alone, the physician should understand that the group A beta-hemolytic streptococcus is the chief *bacterial* cause of pharyngitis in individuals immunized against *C. diphtheriae*. *Chlamydia* and *Mycoplasma* are uncommon causes of pharyngitis in children. Therefore, when one elects to treat pharyngitis in children with an antibiotic, therapy should be directed against the streptococcus and nothing else.

Treatment of streptococcal pharyngitis

The aim of treatment is to prevent rheumatic fever and minimize the chances of spreading the infection to others. To prevent rheumatic fever it is necessary to eradicate the streptococci from the throat, and to achieve eradication we need persistence of the antibiotic in the body for about 10 days. Thus, eradication depends on the choice of drug and the duration of effective blood levels (Table 12.2).

Table 12.2   Streptococcal pharyngitis: antibiotic therapy

Recommended treatment			
Benzathine	<30 kg	600,000 units	
Penicillin G	30–45 kg	900,000 units	Single dose,
	>45 kg	1.2 million units	intramuscularly
Penicillin G or V		250 to 500 mg twice daily	10 days by mouth
Erythromycin (for patients allergic to penicillin)		20–40 mg/kg twice daily	10 days by mouth
Effective but not recommended			
Ampicillin			
Amoxycillin			
Dicloxacillin			
Lincomycin			
Clindamycin			
Cephalosporins			
Not effective or contraindicated			
Sulfonamides			
Tetracyclines			
Chloramphenicol			
Trimethoprim			

Penicillin is the drug of choice, since group A streptococci have remained exquisitely sensitive to this antibiotic. A single injection of benzathine penicillin, 0.6 million units in small children and 1.2 million units in older ones, is the most effective drug because it guarantees adequate blood levels for 10 days – the length of time generally required to eradicate streptococci. The local discomfort at the site of the injection is a small price to pay for safety. If a combination of procaine penicillin and benzathine penicillin is used, the severity of local reactions is greatly reduced.* Streptococcal pharyngitis is uncommon in children under 2 years of age, and virtually never causes rheumatic fever. However, if benzathine penicillin is used in this age group, the upper or mid-lateral thigh is safer than the gluteal region for the site of injection. As noted in the previous chapter, as with any intramuscular injection, care must be taken to avoid injecting into a blood vessel.

Oral penicillin, 250–500 mg twice a day for 10 days, may be used, but there is the risk that the medication will be discontinued when the patient feels better, which is usually in 2–4 days. If one uses oral medication (which does have the advantage that it does not hurt, and that one can

*Studies have shown that a mixture of 900,000 units of benzathine penicillin and 300,000 units of procaine penicillin is a well-tolerated and highly effective preparation in children under 14 years of age. For older children and adults, 1.2 milion units of benzathine penicillin and 300,000 units of procaine penicillin should be used[8].

stop it, should a throat culture turn out to be negative), keep in mind that buffered penicillin G, taken on an empty stomach, seems to be just as effective in the treatment of streptococcal pharyngitis as the more expensive penicillin V or phenoxymethyl penicillin. For patients with a history of penicillin allergy, erythromycin estolate, 20–40 mg/kg twice a day, should be prescribed for 10 days.

The sulfonamides, effective for secondary prevention, should not be used to treat sore throats because they do not eradicate group A streptococci. The tetracyclines, chloramphenicol, and sulfamethoxazole/trimethoprim are ineffective in many cases, or risky, or both. The cephalosporins, ampicillin, and oxacillin are effective against group A streptococci, but no more than penicillin, and are much more costly.

References

1. Fadahuni, H. O. (1981). Rheumatic fever in Nigerian children: A prospective study. *Ann. Trop. Paediatr.*, **1**, 115
2. Denney, F. W. *et al.* (1950). Prevention of rheumatic fever: treatment of the preceding streptococcal infection. *J. Am. Med. Assoc.*, **143**, 151
3. Mohs, E. (1982). Infectious diseases and health care in Costa Rica. *Pediatr. Infect. Dis.*, **1**, 212
4. Gerber, M. A. and Markowitz, M. (1985). Management of streptococcal pharyngitis reconsidered. *Pediatr. Infect. Dis.*, **4**, 518
5. El-Kholy, A. M. *et al.* (1973). A three years' prospective study of streptococcal infections in a population of rural Egyptian school children. *J. Gen. Microbiol.*, **6**, 101
6. El-Batish, M. *et al.* (1985). Streptococcal pharyngitis in Kuwait: A pilot study in the community. *J. Kuwait Med. Assoc.*, **19**, 39
7. Gerber, M. A. *et al.* (1984). Latex agglutination tests for rapid identification of group A streptococci directly from throat swabs. *J. Pediatr.*, **105**, 702
8. Bass, J. W. *et al.* (1976). Streptococcal pharyngitis in children: A comparison of four treatment schedules with intramuscular benzathine penicillin G. *J. Am. Med. Assoc.*, **235**, 1112

Chapter 13
Role of health care workers other than physicians in the control of rheumatic fever

[As Hippocrates wrote] "the physician must not only be prepared to do what is right himself, but also make the patient, the attendants, and the externals cooperate"... he should [therefore] remove the external impediments as much as he can, according to each and every case... only to say what should be done and then to depart, he should not do, because the goal sought will not be attained thereby.

Moses Maimonides, *Commentaries on the Aphorisms of Hippocrates*

There are not enough physicians in most underdeveloped areas to do all the work needed to prevent rheumatic fever, nor is the complex training of a physician truly necessary for many of the tasks. Therefore success depends on the cooperation, effectiveness, and dedication of persons other than physicians: paramedics, physician assistants, nurse practitioners, health program administrators, health educators, teachers, nurses, midwives, house health visitors, school nurses, and village health workers. Most important of all, the potential patients themselves, and their parents, must be reached and become involved. A physician, however, should motivate, educate, and coordinate the others.

When patients have to come long distances to a clinic, inevitably there is a high drop-out rate. The patient with stable, uncomplicated heart disease needs to be seen by a specialist only once, or at the most twice, a year. There would be much less likelihood of non-compliance if the patient could be given his benzathine penicillin injection by a nurse or midwife in the locale where the patient lives or in the school.

It can be argued that rheumatic fever is an occupational disease of schoolchildren. Certainly the school plays a large part in the spreading of streptococcal infection; it should also play a large role in its control.

Where school health services exist they should also be used to identify children with signs suspicious of rheumatic fever. In areas with high prevalence rates of rheumatic heart disease, screening schoolchildren for heart murmurs may be worthwhile. Such screenings may be carried out

Infecções de garganta podem causar
FEBRE REUMÁTICA.

FAÇA ISSO:

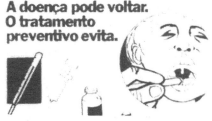

A doença pode voltar.
O tratamento
preventivo evita.

Figure 13.1 A Brazilian poster fostering rheumatic fever prevention (courtesy Dr. Aloysio Ashutti, Belo Horizonte, Brazil)

by physicians or, at less cost, non-physicians trained for this purpose.

To be effective the physician involved in rheumatic fever control should be ready, willing, and able to reach out to the community of physicians and to the larger community of patients, potential patients, and their parents. This reaching out may take the form of a poster (Figure 13.1) or of a health fair (Figure 13.2), of talks to clubs and to associations of parents and teachers, to physicians, to nurses, and in short to anyone who is willing to listen and to some who are not (Figure 13.3).

Primary prevention of rheumatic fever depends on identifying children with "strep throats." Schools are a common locus for the spread of streptococcal infections and are also a good locale for discovering children with these infections. Village health workers are ideally positioned to identify and refer children with acute sore throats for diagnosis and treatment at the local health station.

Health education

Since rheumatic fever is primarily a children's disease, education of parents regarding the importance of treating sore throats to prevent heart disease

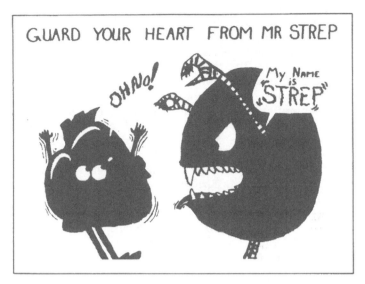

Figure 13.2   Illustration drawn by an elementary school child at a health fair to dramatize the fight between the strep and the patient (courtesy of Dr John Kangos)

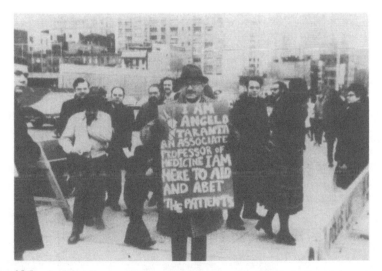

Figure 13.3   A picket line protesting at the closure of a rheumatic fever prevention clinic (Irvington House) joined by one of the authors (A.T.), circa 1970. Usually the proper place of the physician is at the bedside or in the laboratory, but sometimes it's on the picket line

is useful. However, rheumatic fever affects mainly the poor; a difficult-to-reach, often illiterate population. This difficulty could be overcome by television programs in cities where even the lowest socioeconomic population can be reached by TV.

Another way to transmit health information to parents is through their children. Well-designed school programs to teach primary health care issues can make health educators out of elementary school children; this was shown in Central Java, Indonesia, using diarrhea as a model[1]. Since, as this study points out, there are more teachers than health professionals, and more schools than health centers, the school can be an ideal setting for health education, as well as for identifying children with pharyngitis and the early manifestations of rheumatic fever. Health fairs in schools may go a long way towards increasing the "strep-consciousness" of schoolchildren and parents alike.

It is in these related areas of health education and participation of non-physicians in diagnosis and management that inventiveness and a willingness to experiment will pay off the most. Local conditions, of course, will determine the specific approaches to take.

Reference

1. Rohde, J. E. and Sadjimin, T. (1979). Elementary school pupils as health educators: Role of school health programs in primary health care. *Lancet*, **1**, 1350

Chapter 14
The future of rheumatic fever

"It's a poor kind of memory that only works backwards," the Queen remarked.

Lewis Carroll, *Through the Looking Glass*

Futurology is a dangerous vocation; dangerous, that is, to the reputation of futurologists. Nevertheless, the temptation is irresistible to look, however briefly, into the crystal ball.

Streptococcal vaccine

The major obstacles in the development of a streptococcal vaccine have been said to be the multiplicity of streptococcal serotypes and the risk of toxic or allergic reactions[1]. But there has been another deterrent: rheumatic fever had been going away in economically developed countries *without* a vaccine, and the wisdom of the adage prevailed: *if it isn't broken, don't fix it*. However, now that rheumatic fever is staging a comeback in the West, we venture to say that the comeback will stimulate rheumatic fever research, including research on the streptococcal vaccine.

Stimulated largely by the hope of developing an anti-streptococcal vaccine, a considerable amount of work has been done on M proteins, the streptococcal antigens which stimulate type-specific immunity. These proteins have been purified and characterized. They are now recognized as alpha-helical coiled-coil molecules which have been highly purified[2]. But even highly purified M proteins have been associated with an antigenic determinant that is not type-specific and may be responsible for the human hypersensitivity to conventional M protein vaccines[3]. Serum antibody to this non-type-specific M-associated antigen is common in human sera. Fortunately, brief digestion with pepsin greatly reduces the non-type-specific determinants, and isoelectric focusing of an alkaline extract of M protein may have a similar effect[4]. Moreover, chemically synthesized subpeptide fragments of M protein, copying known amino acid sequences of different M proteins, have been found to stimulate type-specific protective immunity *without* stimulating heart cross-reactive antibodies[5,6].

A purified preparation of type 24 M protein extracted with pepsin (pep-M) was shown to be highly immunogenic and free of non-type-specific immunoreactivity. The sequence of the first 29 amino acids was determined

93

and separation from toxic cross-reactive antigens was obtained[7,8]. The purified pep-M was then cleaved with cyanogen bromide, and seven peptides, which together account for the whole amino acid content of the M protein molecule, were purified and characterized. Only the two larger peptides precipitated with type 24 antiserum, but all of them were capable of significantly inhibiting phagocytosis of homologous streptococci in the presence of the same antiserum. Therefore, each of the peptides has the same specific opsonic and presumably protective antigenic determinant. The primary structure of the amino terminal regions of the seven peptides was shown to be markedly similar; therefore pepsin-digested type 24 M protein is composed of repeating covalent structures, which comprise the antigenic determinant responsible for opsonization and type-specific protection[9]. A repetitive subunit structure was also demonstrated by other techniques in type 6 M protein[10].

These important achievements pave the way to the preparation of new, non-toxic streptococcal vaccines for human use, which, we predict, will enter clinical trial soon. However, it is possible that new M types may evolve under the selective pressure of the new immunity induced by vaccines.

Other possible advances

Progress is being made in developing other means to facilitate the prevention of rheumatic fever. One or more B-cell alloantigens are reportedly detectable by monoclonal antibodies in a majority of patients with rheumatic fever[11]. Thus it may become possible to define individuals who are susceptible to rheumatic fever. If this proves indeed to be the case, conventional primary prevention measures could be concentrated only on those who are genetically prone to rheumatic fever.

It may not be too improbable a prediction that the bacterial substances mediating attachment, such as lipoteichoic acid, might be used in the future to competitively inhibit the attachment of bacteria to human cells, or to dislodge them, as a new approach to prevention and to treatment, respectively. Alternatively, antibodies to lipoteichoic acid might be used to block the attachment points of the streptococci.

At a less science-fictional level, methods for the rapid laboratory diagnosis of streptococcal infection are already available and even more reliable methods are likely in the offing. In the treatment of rheumatic fever itself we are also likely to see some new approaches if the disease re-establishes its hold in the West, and relinquishes its status of "orphan disease."

A future without vaccine

It may well be that our crystal ball is cloudy, and a streptococcal vaccine will not be around for a long while. Fortunately, available approaches to the control of rheumatic fever are effective – though they are, no doubt, labor-intensive and "expensive" – and they are effective even in unfavorable social settings. In fact, the effectiveness of secondary prophylaxis, and even of primary prophylaxis, was demonstrated among children of the "inner-city" slums and in military recruits living in crowded barracks, respectively[12,13]. The means of control, therefore, are at hand. But *"ultimately, most health problems that start as scientific problems end up as problems of values that can be solved only by the people themselves and by their representatives. They will have to answer the question, What price human life?"*[14].

References

1. Stollerman, G. H. (1978). Streptococcal immunology: Protection vs. injury. *Ann. Intern. Med.*, **80**, 422
2. Phillips, G. N. Jr *et al.* (1981). Streptococcal M protein: alpha-helical coiled-coil structure and arrangement on the cell surface. *Proc. Natl. Acad. Sci., U.S.A.*, **78**, 4689
3. Beachey, E. H. and Stollerman, G. H. (1972). The common antigen(s) of streptococcal M protein vaccines causing hyperimmune reactions in man. *Trans. Assoc. Am. Phys.*, **85**, 212
4. Cunningham, M. and Beachey, E. H. (1975). Immunochemical properties of streptococcal M protein purified by isoelectric focusing. *J. Immunol.*, **115**, 1002
5. Beachey, E. H. *et al.* (1984). Epitope specific protective immunogenicity of chemically synthesized 12, 18 and 23 residue peptide fragments of streptococcal M protein. *Proc. Natl. Acad. Sci., U.S.A.*, **81**, 2203
6. Beachey, E. H. and Seyer, J. M. (1986). Protective and non-protective epitopes of chemically synthesized peptides of the NH2-terminal region of type 6 streptococcal M protein. *J. Immunol.*, **136**, 2287
7. Beachey, E. H. *et al.* (1977). Purification and properties of M protein extracted from group A streptococci with pepsin: covalent structure of the aminoterminal region of type 24 M antigen. *J. Exp. Med.*, **145**, 1469
8. Beachey, E. H. *et al.* (1977). Separation of the type specific M protein from toxic cross reactive antigens of group A streptococci. *Trans. Assoc. Am. Phys.*, **90**, 390
9. Beachey, E. H. *et al.* (1978). Repeating covalent structure of streptococcal M protein. *Proc. Natl. Acad. Sci., U.S.A.*, **75**, 3163
10. Fischetti, V. A. *et al.* (1976). Streptococcal M protein extracted by nonionic detergent. I. Properties of the antiphagocytic and type-specific molecules. *J. Exp. Med.*, **144**, 32
11. Zabriskie, J. B. *et al.* (1985). Rheumatic fever-associated B cell alloantigens as identified by monoclonal antibodies. *Arthritis Rheum.*, **28**, 1047
12. Wood, H. F. *et al.* (1964). Rheumatic fever in children and adolescents: a long-term epidemiologic study of subsequent prophylaxis, streptococcal infections, and clinical sequelae. III. Comparative effectiveness of three prophylaxis regimens in preventing streptococcal infections and rheumatic recurrences. *Ann. Intern. Med.*, **60** (Feb. Suppl.), 31
13. Wannamaker, L. W. *et al.* (1951). Prophylaxis of acute rheumatic fever by treatment of the preceding streptococcal infection with various amounts of depot penicillin. *Am. J. Med.*, **10**, 673
14. Rheumatic Fever and Rheumatic Heart Disease Study Group, Inter-Society Commission for Heart Disease Resources (1970). Prevention of rheumatic fever and rheumatic heart disease. *Circulation*, **41**, A1–A15

INDEX